How to Build a Healthy Brain

To G. and Nix. Thank you for believing in me.

How to Build a Healthy Brain

Reduce stress, anxiety and depression and future-proof your brain

Kimberley Wilson

First published in Great Britain in 2020 by Yellow Kite
An imprint of Hodder & Stoughton
An Hachette UK company

1

Copyright © 2020 Kimberley Wilson

Illustrations by Rachael Tremlett © Hodder & Stoughton 2020

Illustrations based on Shutterstock images

A CIP catalogue record for this title is available from the British Library

Hardback ISBN 978 1 529 34702 9
eBook ISBN 978 1 529 34851 4

Typeset in Celeste by Hewer Text UK Ltd, Edinburgh
Printed and bound in Great Britain by Clays Ltd, Elcograf S.p.A.

Hodder & Stoughton policy is to use papers that are natural, renewable
and recyclable products and made from wood grown in sustainable
forests. The logging and manufacturing processes are expected to conform
to the environmental regulations of the country of origin.

Yellow Kite
Hodder & Stoughton Ltd
Carmelite House
50 Victoria Embankment
London EC4Y 0DZ

www.yellowkitebooks.co.uk

Contents

Introduction

I grew up with an intimate knowledge of mental illness and neuro-degenerative disease; multiple sclerosis, epilepsy, schizophrenia, motor neurone disease, Guillain-Barré syndrome, borderline person-ality disorder, antisocial personality disorder (sociopathy) and depression all run in my immediate family. This unusual introduc-tion to the darker side of mental life set me apart from my peers. By the time I started school I understood what demyelination was, knew how to spot the signs of an imminent epileptic seizure and could explain the technical definition of psychosis. I understood deeply the fallout, for both individuals and families, when some-thing goes wrong in the brain. But I almost certainly knew too much; I can still remember the rising anxiety I felt whenever I noticed a potential 'symptom' like pins and needles or an unex-plained ringing in my ears. Was this the start? If you have watched the film *It Follows* you will have some idea of what I mean – a nagging sense that something was coming, and that it would get me eventually. Fortunately, I managed to sidestep any serious experi-ence of health anxiety, but, in truth, it was not until I passed through my mid-twenties (75 per cent of psychological disorders develop by the age of 24) that I was able to relax. I was out of the woods.

Thinking back, it is no surprise that I became interested in psychology and mental health. In a bid to understand what was happening in the brains of those around me I embarked on my professional training. At the same time, to do whatever I could to protect my own mental health, I undertook additional training in nutrition and explored the other environmental factors that are known to increase an individual's risk of developing a mental or neurological illness. Psychiatry had long ago abandoned the notion that psychological distress had solely genetic causes, and evidence was growing about the influence of other factors, such as early life stress, previous trauma and nutritional status, on brain (dys)function. I began synthesising that information into regular habits and principles that I could apply to my own life and those of my friends and family.

During my final year of training a study was published that made quite a splash in the field of psychiatry. Felice Jacka, an Australian epidemiologist, had found a correlation between overall diet quality and mental health in women. Women who had healthier diets – higher in fruit and vegetables, wholegrains, fish and unprocessed meat – were less prone to anxiety and depression. These common mental health concerns are the central focus of every psychologist's training and, with my own interest in food, lifestyle and risk reduction, I continued to closely follow this area of research (now called Nutritional Psychiatry).

After qualifying and becoming a Chartered Psychologist I began my career in what was then Europe's largest women's prison, HMP & YOI Holloway in north London. Around this time a Dutch study was published replicating the findings of a previous British study that showed that male prisoners were significantly less aggressive when they were provided with nutritional supplements (vitamins, minerals and essential fats) compared to a placebo. This was an incredibly important outcome with profound implications for prisons, prisoners and the criminal justice system. Knowing that aggressive behaviour (including acts of violence against others, self-harm and suicide attempts) was a major safety, staffing and financial concern for the prison, it seemed reasonable to consider improving the (very poor) quality of the food in the establishment, or looking into supplementation, to see whether there would be any effect on violence and aggression. Unfortunately, my efforts did not lead anywhere.

When I stopped working for the prison service and established my own clinic, I decided that I could at least make this valuable information available for my clients. Food and lifestyle have profound effects on brain health, mood and behaviour. This, I believe, is public health information that *everyone* should know.

As a psychologist with my own clinical practice, and from my own history, I see the terrible damage that psychological illnesses can wreak. I have committed myself to helping my clients to recover and reclaim their lives from these conditions, but over the years I have found myself increasingly frustrated by two things:

1. For many people therapy simply isn't enough – mental health is influenced by so many important lifestyle factors that occur outside of the consulting room.

2. Even when I can make people aware of these other issues, I can only see one person for one hour at a time. What about all the people on waiting lists or who haven't yet made it to the doctor to ask for help?

I realised that there is a big gap between what scientists are discovering and what the public is being told about the power we have to influence the impact of these illnesses. There is also little awareness of the importance of taking care of our brains more generally, not just to prevent illness but to improve performance, including having better attention, faster reaction times and improved memory.

This book is designed to bridge those gaps. I want to help you understand that brain health should be a priority for us all and that there are practical habits and exercises you can start using *right now* that will help to improve your brain health and function. In this book I will outline the best available evidence for how you can modify your own lifestyle to improve brain health and reduce your risk of cognitive decline.

Don't wait

One of the most common mistakes that people make in relation to managing their emotional and mental health is waiting until there is a crisis before they act. In part because of the stigma that still pervades mental illness, along with the limited availability of evidence-based, practical information, people feel that they should just 'push through'. But that's the equivalent of waiting for your teeth to fall out before making an appointment with the dentist.

How to Build a Healthy Brain is my manifesto advocating for the practice of *prevention* in mental health in the same way that we do for physical health conditions. Fortunately, many of the habits that help to promote physical wellness – such as safeguarding sleep, engaging in regular physical activity and eating nutrient-dense foods – also support mental health and resilience. Doing what you can to adopt some of these practices is a great start. However, there are also important differences. Much of our psychological health relates to our capacity to understand and manage our emotions and the quality of our relationships – features of mental health that receive too little attention. This book outlines the evidence base for which psychological activities and attitudes have been shown to protect mental health and reduce the risk of mental illness, and provides practical, actionable steps to help you get started.

How To Use This Book:

The chapter 'A Quick Note on Research' is designed to help you navigate your way through the myriad health claims in the media, giving you the skills to tell fact from fiction. 'Getting to Know the Brain' is a whistle stop tour of the brain and neuroanatomy, that will help you get the most out of this book. If you want to get straight to the good stuff you can go directly to Chapter 4.

I begin by introducing the two crucial aspects of brain health. I call these the 'major players'. Balancing these two factors is the key to tipping the balance in favour of better brain function, both in the short- and long-term. From there each chapter describes how individual lifestyle habits control or influence the major players. By the end of the book you will understand the best-known risk factors for brain health and will have discovered how to reduce or reverse them. Each chapter ends with a list of practical 'takeaways' – tips and actions that you can start to implement immediately – and there are also a few quick questionnaires along the way. These will allow you to assess where you currently are in your process of building a healthy brain, and where there are areas for improvement.

Dementia does not have to be an inevitable part of ageing. In fact, a paper published in 2019 found that older people who followed healthy lifestyle advice, as outlined in this book, had a 30 per cent reduced risk of developing dementia, even when they carried genes that put them at higher risk. And there is no need for expensive superfood powders or mountain retreats; most of these effective tools don't cost any money and take very little time.

Taking mental health prevention seriously means being *proactive* in establishing practices that can reduce the risk of psychological decline, addressing stress as soon as possible, and avoiding substances and activities that harm the brain. This book presents some of the latest and strongest evidence available about how to do that. However, it is important to note that risk reduction is not the same as risk *elimination*. A percentage of what happens to our health is down to luck. Some people can live pristine life-styles and still develop illness. Nonetheless, the science is clear that we can reduce our risk of developing common mental health concerns, such as depression and Alzheimer's disease, by adjusting lifestyle behaviours and the more people adopt protective habits the more they will stave off or delay developing these illnesses.

Having a healthy brain is the key to enjoying a full and satisfy-ing life, increasing our abilities, performance, creativity and our sense of life satisfaction. Throughout this book I hope to empower you with both the *why* and the *how* of better brain health and emotional resilience. I want to help you to have a stronger, more resilient brain, so turn the page and let's get started!

CHAPTER 1

The Global Burden
of Mental Illness

There is a great deal of discussion in the media about the rise in non-communicable or 'lifestyle' diseases and the urgent need for effective policies and treatments to end this trend. But which disease is the leading cause of disability across the world? Diabetes? Heart disease? These are both good guesses. But the answer is actually depression. This means that more people suffer impairments in daily functioning – such as attending school and work, and enjoying social relationships – because of depression than illnesses like cancer or stroke. In only 10 years depression will be the *leading* cause of global disease burden – a measure of how much an illness affects quality of life, life expectancy and the economy.

Depression is a term for a group of overlapping symptoms that together significantly impair a person's mood and ability to function. Depression is often thought to be solely an illness of the brain, but it actually leaves its mark throughout the body and is characterised by a range of psychological, physical and interpersonal symptoms:

Psychological

- persistent low mood or sadness
- feelings of hopelessness and helplessness
- low motivation
- loss of interest in things that were formerly pleasurable
- low self-esteem
- tearfulness
- feelings of guilt
- irritability
- impaired decision-making
- anxiety
- thoughts of self-harm or suicide

Physical

- sleep disturbance
- appetite or weight changes
- gut symptoms
- lack of energy
- slow movements and/or speech
- aches and pains
- loss of libido
- changes to the menstrual cycle
- self-neglect

Interpersonal

- poor functioning or performance at school or work
- social withdrawal
- relationship difficulties

We have had effective drug treatments for depression since the late 1950s so why is depression a growing global problem? Frustratingly, our current modes of treatment (typically antidepressant medication and/or talking therapy) are not as effective or accessible as we need them to be. As the number of people being diagnosed with depression has grown, so have the prescriptions for antidepressants. Yet more than half the people taking antidepressants in the UK have ongoing symptoms. This discrepancy between the first-line treatments and residual symptoms has led to a rethink about what causes depression and, therefore, how it should be treated. It's not that medication is not a valuable tool, but perhaps we have been so focused on it that we have forgotten to check what else might be in the toolbox. On top of this, across the country, mental health departments are short-staffed, services are being closed and helplines shut down, meaning that talking therapy, an effective treatment for depression, is inaccessible for a growing number of patients.

There is now robust evidence from human trials that certain lifestyle factors – our daily habits and activities – can help to prevent depression from developing or reduce its severity. Many of these factors are cheap, or free, and can be implemented immediately. I have written this book to give you access to this research and practical tools to turn the evidence into easy, everyday habits.

Young people

In Western countries depression is directly linked to the second largest cause of death in young people. After accidents, the major cause of loss of life in those aged 15–29 is suicide, which is typically driven by depression. Sadly, rates of depression and suicide in young people have increased faster over the last 15 years than at any point since records began. There are some important questions being asked about what has caused this sudden rise in the levels of distress that young people are experiencing. The answer appears to be a combination of environmental, social and lifestyle factors that undermine physical brain health and psychological resilience. We will take a closer look at several of these factors throughout this book.

Older adults

What about later in life? In the last few years, dementia (including Alzheimer's disease) became the leading cause of death in the UK. In 2017 the World Health Organization estimated that there were 47 million people living with dementia across the world. By 2030 that figure will jump to 75 million. A new case is diagnosed every three seconds.

Dementia is the name for a group of devastating age-related neurodegenerative disorders. In these illnesses, over a period of many years, brain cells begin to break down and die, creating lesions (gaps) in the brain tissue. The sufferer progressively loses cognitive function, particularly in domains such as memory and decision-making. There is currently no cure for dementia. In fact, some of the world's largest drug companies recently abandoned development of dementia drugs due to lack of efficacy in clinical trials. Again, this is leading many in the field of neuroscience to re-evaluate previous assumptions about the causes of dementia, opening up new avenues for research and intervention.

That said, in the world of medicine it is already common knowledge that dementia *is not an inevitable part of ageing*. A recent review by *The Lancet*, one of the world's most respected scientific research journals, estimated that, if we carefully followed the best lifestyle advice, we could prevent up to a third of global cases of Alzheimer's. That translates to up to 15 million fewer people being struck down by this terrible disease.

If one in three cases of Alzheimer's disease could be prevented or delayed with improvements to lifestyle and daily habits, why isn't this crucial information easily available to the public? Why don't more people know about it? A recent survey found that while nearly half (42 per cent) of UK adults say that dementia is the disease they fear most, only 34 per cent thought that you could reduce your risk and only 1 per cent could name the seven known risk factors (smoking, high blood pressure, diabetes, obesity, depression, lack of mental stimulation and physical inactivity). The lack of committed and comprehensive investment in a public health campaign for the brain leaves our communities even more vulnerable to these life-shattering illnesses.

The Growing Mental Health Crisis

There is a long history of the brain and mental health being short-changed in comparison to physical health. Despite being some of the most significant causes of disease burden in the world, mental health research is still woefully underfunded. I know from personal experience as the former manager of a National Health Service (NHS) mental health facility that, when budgets are cut, mental health provisions are first in line for the chop.

When we look at the prevalence of mental illness, the growing rates of diagnosis, the restrictions on access to treatment and the protracted recovery, this 'mental-health-last' approach makes very little sense. A report by one of the UK's largest mental health charities found that 40 per cent of visits to a general practitioner (GP) involve mental health concerns. A separate NHS report showed that mental illness (including anxiety and stress) is the number one reason people take sickness leave from work and, when they do, they are off for longer periods than for physical conditions.

This wide-scale favouring of physical health over mental health also ignores the fact that mental health conditions often have significant physical symptoms, as listed on page 8. This means that when someone goes to their GP for stomach problems, back pain or fatigue, both doctor and patient may be erroneously engaged in looking for a physical cause for an illness when it is in fact a psychological one. Failing to hold the brain in mind causes delays in identifying the true cause, and the right treatment, for many patients.

One of the reasons for the disparity between how mental health conditions are treated in comparison to physical illness is the erroneous belief that mental health conditions are not 'real', that they are solely a problem of psychology and not biology. It's so important to remember that the brain is an organ; it's just an incredibly complicated one with some very special functions. For example, we all know that for our heart to work properly we have to look after it by eating well, exercising, avoiding smoking, and so on. A heart that is not properly cared for will begin to show impairments in its function through changes in blood pressure, palpitations and pain. These are the clues that our heart needs some extra attention. The same principle applies to the brain. A brain that is struggling will begin to show impairments in its functions; it just so happens that the brain's functions are mood, personality, planning, decision-making, information processing and memory. These are the clues that the brain needs some extra attention, but too many people brush these symptoms off as incidental or, worse, something to be ashamed of and ignored.

The idea that mental illness is somehow 'less real' than physical illness doesn't make us stronger. In fact, quite the opposite. We know that recovery from mental health conditions is best if you intervene as early as possible, during the first episode or when symptoms are mild. However, the misunderstanding and stigma around mental illness means that people sit on their symptoms of brain distress for weeks, months, and sometimes years. By the time the symptoms are bad enough for them to seek professional help, the illness is much more entrenched and more difficult to treat.

It is, unfortunately, no exaggeration to say that we a facing a global mental and brain health crisis. I cannot state this more clearly: across the lifespan, from the young to the elderly, *the leading causes of death and disability are illnesses of the brain and mental health.* As well as the rise in depression, in the UK there was a 14 per cent increase in Alzheimer's deaths between 2016 and 2017. And scientists have dismissed the suggestion that this is simply because we are living longer: not only are more people affected, but these conditions are affecting people earlier in their lives than ever before. Alongside this the number of people living with severe mental illness is growing; more people are being detained under the Mental Health Act and around 1 in 10 children now has a diagnosable mental health condition. Something is profoundly wrong. There is something – or many things – about the way that we are living, the way that we are neglecting our brain health, that is putting us all at greater risk. For me, it is simply not enough to say that someone is depressed or that they have insufficient serotonin available in the brain. These statements are descriptive but they don't tell us anything about *why* this is happening and, importantly, what we might be able to do about it – how we get to the root cause of this dysregulation.

How to Build a Healthy Brain brings together the latest research on the known, modifiable risk factors for mental illness and neurodegeneration, helps you to understand the science and empowers you with effective, practical tools to start improving and protecting your brain health today and for years to come.

CHAPTER 2

A Quick Note on Research

It is impossible to open a newspaper or read an article nowadays without coming across a piece of apparently groundbreaking health research that claims to extend or enhance your life. If a lot of the time that information seems contradictory, that's because it is, but that usually isn't the fault of the researchers; it's down to the new way that we consume our news.

In the 'olden days' (before the year 2000!) newspapers and a handful of TV news programmes had the monopoly on how we acquired our information. All news had to be accessed from a finite number of daily editions or broadcasts. If a news story broke after the *Ten O'Clock News* or the evening edition it might appear on the radio but otherwise we all had to wait until the next publication cycle to find out what happened. On top of that, these outlets had a small number of gatekeepers; editors or science journalists who had the final say on what got written about and published.

As the world moved into the digital era that old model started to fade away. News websites could be updated in seconds and a deluge of dedicated news channels suddenly had hours of airtime to fill. This technological shift caused a change in the function of news: where in the past the news was a 'service', today it is better described as a 'market'. Most of the major news websites are funded by advertising, a revenue model that depends on capturing as many eyes as possible. In this highly competitive news market clicks mean everything, so editors have to find a way to make their content as compelling as possible. Psychologically, the best way to capture someone's attention is to appeal to their emotions and, because we evolved to rapidly respond to threat, editors spin headlines to create as dramatic-sounding a story as possible.

I have spoken to many researchers and journalists who felt unhappy about the headline that was applied to their study or story. It is also very common for research that has only been conducted on mice or even on cells in a cell culture dish to be published as though the results apply to humans. Often you have to read through several paragraphs (most people don't) to discover that the story pertains to a mouse mother fed large amounts of caffeine and not human mothers drinking coffee, for example.

For their part, the editors are simply doing their jobs – getting as many people as they can to click on their story, securing revenue for the company. However, the result for the consumer is an unhelpfully confusing array of dramatic news stories with advice that seemingly changes by the hour. This doesn't just leave the reader unsure of what to believe, it makes us doubt the validity of scientific research altogether. This is, of course, hugely unfair on the researchers who work hard to conduct high-quality research, but also does a disservice to the public who rely on these outlets to translate and disseminate the gems of really useful information hidden within hard-to-access scientific journals or overshadowed by a sensationalist headline.

The role of social media

There has been another addition to the information landscape
that makes navigating the health and wellness space even more
perilous: social media. Social media platforms such as Twitter,
Facebook and Instagram have fundamentally changed the way
we consume information. For the most part this is of huge benefit to humanity. The speed with which stories, videos and peti-
tions can now be shared has provided new outlets for social
justice activism, disaster intervention and financial aid. It has
also changed the way in which we access health information with
people turning to bloggers and lifestyle influencers for their
health information. A recent PWC Health Institute report found
that 90 per cent of young people believe the health information
they find on social media. However, unlike registered health
professionals, many of these people are unqualified, have not
been taught to read and interpret scientific data, and are not
bound by professional codes of ethics and practice. This means
that, even with the best intentions, they may be disseminating
unreliable or false information to their hundreds, thousands,
perhaps millions of followers.

Following bad health advice can have serious consequences.
Wellness blogger Belle Gibson was able to amass thousands of
followers and hundreds of thousands of dollars falsely claiming
that she had cured terminal brain cancer with a plant-based diet.
Who knows how many vulnerable people followed her example
before the truth came out? Thousands of social media accounts
promote a range of health 'treatments' for which there is absolutely no scientific evidence, such as the alkaline diet for cancer or
celery juice as a panacea. In 2018 an American court awarded $105
million in damages to a woman who was encouraged to eschew

conventional cancer treatment in favour of an 'alkaline-based' treatment. Her illness is now terminal.

Fortunately, increasing numbers of researchers and healthcare professionals are now taking to posting their research directly on their own social media pages, allowing them to explain exactly what they found, what it means and to whom it should relate. This was the reason that I decided to move my own social media presence away from the occasional picture of my lunch to a mental health resource where I explain and share research on mental health, psychology and Nutritional Psychiatry. Increasingly, publications and influencers are seeking out the advice and opinions of qualified experts, which will help to reduce confusion and keep consumers safe. That said, it is also important that consumers are able to think critically about the information they are presented with and what someone means by 'evidence'.

Not All Research is Created Equal

The scientific method attempts to refine our notions of 'truth' by testing assumptions under rigorous conditions, and there is an established process to move from an idea (hypothesis) to accepted knowledge and treatment. Let's imagine I am an eighteenth-century doctor called Edward Jenner and I have a hypothesis that people who have previously been exposed to cowpox (found in cattle) develop immunity to smallpox. Smallpox was at the time a highly contagious and deadly viral disease (happily it has since been eradicated through successful vaccination programmes) and it would be extremely valuable to understand whether being infected with the milder cowpox virus could protect people against the more dangerous small-pox. As the person proposing the hypothesis, in strict scientific practice, it is my responsibility to disprove it. The scientific method tasks me with doing everything that I can to prove myself wrong and, if I cannot, then I can say that my hypothesis is supported. Notice that I didn't say 'proven'. This is because there is always the chance that there is a piece of contradictory or interfering information out there that I (or others) haven't yet come across. In this way the scientific method always leaves room for new and better evidence.

If you have read any scientific articles yourself, or have listened to interviews with researchers, you will have heard the speakers use a lot of language that makes it seem as though they are unsure of what they are saying. The results always 'suggest' or 'indicate' that an idea 'may' be 'supported'. It may sound as though these scientists are hedging their bets but this language is actually a reflection of scientific rigor and intellectual honesty. They will be confident of what they found but the principles of the scientific method mean they are leaving space for the outcomes to be refined by future research.

Not all evidence carries equal weight when it comes to quality, authority and generalisability. In evidence-based medicine (EBM) the 'hierarchy of evidence', usually depicted as a pyramid, ranks the quality and strength of scientific evidence:

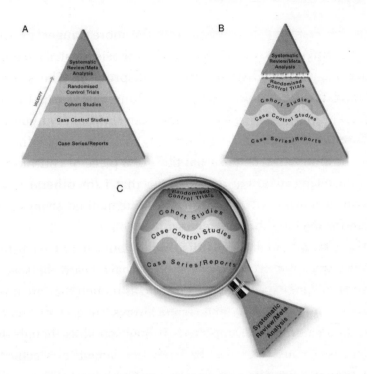

(Source: Murad, M. H., Asi, N., Alsawas, M. and Alahdab, F., 2016. New evidence pyramid. *BMJ Evidence-Based Medicine*, 21(4), pp.125–7)

Case reports

At the base of the pyramid are case reports – observations from individual practitioners on individual patients/cases. They are often interesting to read because an experienced clinician is in a good position to notice unexpected or novel outcomes of a treatment or intervention, cases that buck the trend or contradict the current paradigm. However, because case reports relate to individual observations that have simply emerged in a one-off situation, they cannot account for any unique factors of the practitioner, patient or environment that might have an influence on what is being observed. For example, what if whatever is being observed was just an accident? Case reports can help us to develop hypotheses that can be rigorously tested higher up the pyramid.

Mechanism studies

In *in vitro* studies, cell or tissue samples are exposed to the substance being tested. So I might take some human immune cells and expose them to the cowpox virus. I could then test how these immune cells respond when they are later exposed to smallpox. If they were able to fend off the smallpox virus I would have my first piece of evidence that, at least on a cellular level, there was a relationship between cowpox exposure and smallpox immunity. But events that occur on a cellular level do not always translate on a systems level. Systems are much more complex than individual cell activity and there could be hundreds of other factors in a system that interfere with the action we have observed in the cell culture dish.

Animal models

Animal models give researchers a clearer sense of the nature of the interaction between an active compound and a live biological system. Commonly, experiments will be conducted with mice or rats that have been specially bred to exhibit a murine (mouse or rat) version of a human illness such as Alzheimer's disease or multiple sclerosis. Animal research illuminates the biological mechanisms that might be involved in a disease action when it is not possible to conduct the research with human participants.

It is worth saying that scientists have to apply for stringent ethical permission before they start conducting experiments with animals. In their ethics applications researchers have to clearly explain how they will care for the animals and demonstrate that they have considered all ways in which they will limit the animal's distress during the trial.

At the top of the pyramid are randomised controlled trials, systematic reviews and meta-analyses.

Randomised controlled trials

Randomised controlled trials (RCTs) are considered the gold standard in EBM research because of their ability to reduce the opportunity for bias within the study protocol, and for quantifying whether a drug or intervention is more effective than doing nothing, administering a placebo or regression to the mean (the tendency for most unusual results to drift back to normal levels without intervention). Typically, in an RCT participants are randomly allocated to either the active arm of the trial (where they receive the real treatment) or the placebo condition (an identical but inactive intervention). For example, 100 people volunteer to participate in a vaccination trial. Fifty will be randomly allocated to receive the vaccine and 50 will get the placebo, such as an injection of saline that will have no effect on immunity. Importantly, neither group will know whether they are getting the real treatment or not, and ideally neither would the nurse administering the injections. They are then exposed to the live virus and assessed for how many from each group go on to develop the infection.

At this stage researchers are in a position to say whether one thing *causes* or has a direct effect on another in particular groups of people.

What if we're not testing a drug? When it comes to lifestyle habits it is incredibly difficult to prevent people knowing whether they are in the active or placebo condition of the trial, especially in nutrition studies. Researchers in these fields have to work incredibly hard to design RCTs appropriate to what is being studied.

Also, when studying lifestyle, we can make the general assumption that the activity or behaviours (e.g. exercise) are not toxic, therefore rather than safety, lifestyle intervention trials will look at efficacy; what combination of which behaviours over what period of time will have a positive or negative effect on a target health outcome?

Systematic reviews and meta-analyses

Evidence from RCTs can tell us about causality but, strictly, results are still confined to the population on which it was tested. It is not uncommon, for example, for research to be conducted on small groups of a particular population, such as white, male university students. This is often an opportunity sample (most research labs are parts of universities) but it means that researchers risk overlooking features that are specific to women or people of other ethnicities, for example.

Systematic reviews and meta-analyses allow the results of several small trials to be pooled together to look for overall trends. This can give us more confidence that the results that were observed can be generalised to large populations rather than small idiosyncratic groups. This is, of course, really important when making recommendations at a national or population level.

You're in charge

I have heard it said that patients and the public do not need to be given the evidence when it comes to health information – they just need to be told what to do. I strongly disagree with this position for a few reasons:

1. I think it's insulting. This kind of attitude underestimates an individual's willingness and ability to understand why they are being advised to change their behaviour and what outcomes they can expect.

2. It's based on the 'argument from authority' (also known as the 'appeal to authority'). This is a kind of poor reasoning that says, 'You should do as I say because I am an authority.' However, simply being an authority (e.g. having the right qualifications) doesn't automatically make someone's information or practice sound. (There are plenty of examples of doctors struck off for malpractice that demonstrate this.) Instead, I believe that, rather than appealing to authority, professionals in all fields should be supporting greater public engagement with science communication and campaigning for higher standards of science reporting in the media. We should be skilling more people up, not dumbing the information down.

3. Psychologically, that is not how people work. Sure, there are some individuals who have an innate tendency to be more compliant and will be content to simply do as they are told. But most people have a strong need for autonomy, and to feel that they have power and choice over their own behaviours. On top of that, change that is made to satisfy an intrinsic authority rather than an external one is more durable.

Takeaways

- Science is a methodology that attempts to get closer and closer to an objective, robust 'truth' while always leaving space for the things that are not yet known.
- There is a hierarchy of evidence. Broadly speaking, the higher up the hierarchy one goes the more difficult and expensive the research is to conduct, but the more confident we can be of the conclusions.
- When you read a news headline or a blog post about a health claim look for what level of evidence is being reported. If possible, ask the person to provide a link to the source they are referring to. It is not enough that the person 'seems trustworthy' or has a large online following. When it comes to implementing advice that could have an effect on your health you deserve to have the best quality, most reliable information you can get.
- The research I refer to in this book is based on human trials, because I want the information to be as relevant to you as possible. Where I mention animal trials this will be clearly identified and used in relation to explaining a mechanism of action where it is not possible or ethical to conduct the research with human participants.

CHAPTER 3

Getting to Know the Brain

Imagine you are walking down the street listening to music. Your brain is interpreting the information coming in from your eyes about the conditions of the pavement. Is it gravel or paved? Is there a lamp post coming up that you need to avoid? It is then coordinating this information with the sensory data coming in from your feet and legs, and making judgements about how much pressure to apply to the ground, and how and when to bend or extend your knees. Specialised areas of your brain will be holding in mind your destination and what you expect to happen when you get there. At the same time the tiny vibrations created by the soundwaves as they hit your eardrums are translated into electrical signals that will be further interpreted into music or words. Receptors in your skin relay information about the air temperature and your brain makes a decision about whether you should button up your coat or take off your scarf to help regulate your internal body temperature.

At the same time a vast network of messages are being exchanged about other important internal conditions. The relative availability of water or glucose in the blood will translate into a conscious awareness of thirst or hunger. The accumulation of certain molecules in the brain translates into varying degrees of alertness or a desire to sleep. Interoception – the perception of what is happening inside the body – will indicate hunger, satiety or the need to pee.

This activity doesn't stop when you close your eyes and go to sleep, far from it. As your brain moves through the different levels of sleep (see page 69 for more on this) it begins the nightly process of reorganising the events of the day. Important details and information are encoded while insignificant ones are archived or allowed to fade. Furthermore, during sleep your brain undergoes a deep clean, clearing away the accumulated debris of the day, helping to keep your brain healthy.

The human brain is the most complex structure in the known universe. This is why it always astounds me when people expect themselves to completely understand their own minds. Most people don't understand their phones, so why would you expect yourself to understand an organ that is many hundreds of times more complex? Nonetheless, it will be helpful for you to know a little bit of neuroanatomy to get the most out of this book. That way, as you move through the chapters, you will have a better sense of the physical actions that all the tips and habits are exerting on your brain. And you will better understand why it is all so important.

Brain Cells

Motor Neurone

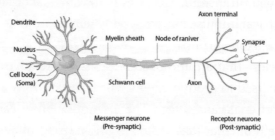

At The Synapse

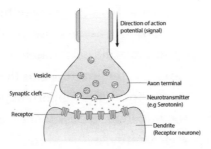

As the action potential travels along the axon, it triggers vesicles (sacs containing the neurotransmitter) to fuse with the synaptic membrane. The neurotransmitter is released and drifts across the synaptic cleft where some dock to receptors, triggering a new action potential. Some of the neurotransmitter drifts back to the presynaptic neurone where it is replaced/re-uptaken.

There are several types of cell in the brain, each playing an important and complementary role to the other. The type of cell that most people are familiar with is the nerve cell or 'neurone'. Neurones are couriers in the brain system; they are responsible for relaying messages to and from the brain and the body.

Neurones have a 'soma' or cell body that contains the nucleus. The nucleus contains the cell's DNA – the packet of information that tells the cell what to do. The branch-like projections, 'dendrites', receive the information from the preceding cell in the form of chemicals called neurotransmitters that initiate an electrical impulse.

This electrical impulse ('action potential') travels down the axon towards the axon terminal. Within the axon terminal are sacs, called 'vesicles', that are filled with the neurotransmitter that the cell is specialised to produce. The arrival of the action potential at the axon terminal causes the vesicles to move towards the edge ('membrane') of the axon terminal. There it fuses with the membrane and releases the neurotransmitter into the space between the axon terminal of the first cell and the dendrite of the next one. This space is referred to as the 'synaptic cleft' or 'synapse'.

The neurotransmitter molecules drift across the synapse and connect with receptors on the dendrites of the post-synaptic neurone. When the neurotransmitter binds with the receptor it triggers an action potential in the axon of the post-synaptic neurone and the process continues.

The axon can be thought of as a wire or cable, sending an electrical signal from one end to the other. Similarly, the axon is insulated (like the plastic around your household wires). The insulation around an axon is a fat-based substance called 'myelin', which helps to increase the speed at which the action potential travels down the axon.

Glia

Glia are brain cells that do not send messages but help to protect and support the function of neurones. Some types of glia are astrocytes, oligodendrocytes and microglia. I'll just highlight a couple of their functions as they will be relevant later on.

Astrocytes One of the main functions of astrocytes is maintaining the physical shape of the brain, but they are also important for the development and survival of neurones and can increase the strength and activity of synapses, as well as their overall development. Astrocytes feed neurones by extracting nutrients from the blood and passing them to neurones. They are also able to produce glucose, the preferred form of energy for nerve cells.

Oligodendrocytes This type of glial cell produces two proteins called brain-derived neurotrophic factor (BDNF) and insulin-like growth factor-1 (IGF-1). These proteins promote the growth of new neurones and connections (synapses) and support the survival of the ones we already have. This is hugely important because, as you will come to see, protecting the brain cells we already have is the best hope we have of securing long-term brain health.

In the brain and spinal cord oligodendrocytes produce the myelin that wraps around the axon.

Microglia Microglia make up about 15 per cent of the brain and play an important role in the brain's immune response. Microglia have long branches that stretch out and monitor the conditions around nearby nerve cells. When they notice a problem one of the things they do is engulf or 'eat' harmful agents within the brain, such as bacteria from an infection (a process called 'phagocytosis').

They are also able to fight off unwanted pathogens by releasing powerful toxic chemicals. However, if this process goes unchecked these chemicals can actually harm neurones. We'll talk about the circumstances under which this happens in Chapter 5.

When they are activated by the presence of bacteria, a virus or a brain injury, the microglia multiply and release compounds called 'cytokines'. Cytokines are the group name for a number of different proteins that play a crucial role in our immune system's response to illness or injury. When the threat is controlled, the microglia signal for the start of repair processes to fix the damage that has occurred.

The blood–brain barrier
The membranes around most body cells and the lining of blood vessels are partially permeable, which means that they allow water and some other molecules through. This allows the water you

drink to pass through the blood vessels and reach the dehydrated cells in your fingertips, for example. These partially permeable membranes are like the friendly doormen at a nightclub; they'll check your ID and let you through.

Your brain, however, is incredibly selective about what it allows in. Instead of a friendly doorman, the tight junctions of the blood–brain barrier (BBB) are more like a fingerprint scanner at an exclusive private members' club. Only the elite few can gain entry.* This exclusivity means that even cells that form part of the body's immune system can't get through. This is one of the reasons why the brain has developed its own immune defence system in the form of microglia. This selectiveness is essential because the brain is so important and vulnerable to damage that you do not want to risk exposing it to anything that might cause harm.

If something happens in the body that impairs the function of the BBB there may be many negative consequences:

- Interference with the action potential of neurones. Depending on what part of the brain is affected this could contribute to impairments in thinking or movement.
- Immune cells from the body's immune system can get into the brain. Since this is not where they belong this can create a lot of confusion. Either they can mistakenly attack healthy brain tissue, or the brain's own immune cells will attack them. Sometimes both. If this happens the brain may end up in a state of 'neuroinflammation', which is associated with a number of brain diseases and mental health disorders.

---

* There are a handful of important exceptions to this, which are discussed on page 233.

Neural networks

Groups of cells that work together for a particular process form a 'neural circuit' or 'neural network'. These neural networks are like different neighbourhoods in a city. For example, trying to remember where you left your keys will trigger action in a separate network than when you are trying to learn dance moves.

The Prefrontal Cortex

We live in a world that highly prizes thoughts and reason and thinks much less of emotion. 'Being emotional' is another way of saying that someone is being irrational or that they are not thinking correctly. However, from a psychological perspective it does not make sense to try to conceive of thought as distinct from feeling. In fact, it doesn't even make sense biologically when we look at the physical structure of the brain.

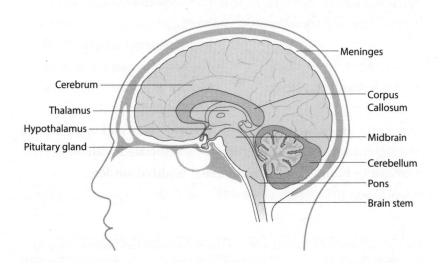

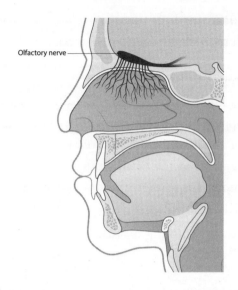

Olfactory nerve

In this image the front section of the brain is the prefrontal cortex (PFC). The relative size of the PFC in humans is the feature that most distinguishes our brains from those of other primates and is understood to give rise to most 'human' capabilities: planning, decision-making, risk assessment, understanding cause and effect, impulse control, social interaction, personality, IQ and much more.

The Limbic System

The limbic area of the brain is associated with emotion processing and regulation. As you can see, not only are these two areas situated next to each other but the frontal region of the limbic lobe actually comprises part of the PFC. *Your emotions are part of your higher psychological functions.* More than that, emotions are a crucial part of our ability to reason, including making decisions.

Taking care of your brain health includes taking your emotions seriously and learning how to understand and respond to them. I discuss this in more detail in Chapter 11.

The hippocampus

You will be reading a lot about this area of the brain throughout the book. The hippocampus can be thought of as the seat of memory as it is crucial for the assimilation and retention of information. It is one of the key areas of the brain damaged in Alzheimer's disease. The hippocampus sits within an area of the brain important for emotion regulation, in which it also plays an important role.

The amygdala

Another core structure of the limbic system, the amygdala is the brain's threat detection centre. For example, people with a diagnosis of generalised anxiety disorder tend to have a larger amygdala, which is linked to paying greater attention to threatening or fearful stimuli.

The hypothalamus

This multitasking area is about the size of an almond in the adult brain and plays important functions for hormone production, sleep regulation, food intake, the stress response and maintenance of body temperature.

Neurological characteristics of common brain disorders

Generalised anxiety disorder (GAD) While we all experience nervousness or anxiety from time to time, a diagnosis of GAD describes the frequent experience of being overwhelmed by anxious thoughts and worries to the degree that it prevents you from being able to enjoy a normal life.

A consistent finding in neuroimaging is that people with a diagnosis of GAD tend to have more grey matter (cell bodies) in their amygdala than non-anxious individuals. They also have more activity in this region, which correlates to symptom severity. The PFC plays a role in how we process threat, and this area seems to be overactive in people with GAD. There is also evidence of decreased grey matter in the hippocampus, and less connectivity between the PFC and the limbic system. Generally, there is a pattern of dysregulation in response to emotion-laden facial expressions and anxiety-inducing stimuli.

Major depressive disorder (MDD, clinical depression or depression) A general finding in people with depressive disorders is that hippocampal volumes and rates of cell growth are lower in people with depression. The change in hippocampal size is understood to be mediated by stress because BDNF production is suppressed by stress. When followed over three years, for example, the brains of people with depression showed declines in brain matter. People with depression also tend to have suboptimal connectivity in the PFC and regions of the brain that are associated with emotion, reward processing and theory of mind, which is our capacity to understand that others have different thoughts, beliefs and ideas from us. These structural and functional differences are thought to account for the cognitive symptoms of depression, such as difficulties concentrating, impaired decision-making, loss of pleasure, lack of motivation and social withdrawal.

Anxiety and MDD are often comorbid, which means they frequently show up together. One theory is that, for some people, the depression emerges as a result of the chronic stress of the anxiety. Correspondingly, the brains of patients with depression show larger grey matter volumes in the amygdala, and the severity of the illness seems to correlate with the change in amygdala volume.

Alzheimer's disease The brains of people with Alzheimer's are characterised by the presence of clumps of a misfolded protein called 'amyloid beta', which accumulates in the synapse and interferes with signalling between the nerves. There is also the presence of tangles of 'tau', another protein that aggregates within the cell, disrupting cell function and eventually causing the neurone to collapse. After a while, when many cells have been affected, lesions appear in the brain, particularly in the hippocampus, leading to the signature memory impairments of the disease.

There has recently been a shift in the scientific understanding of what causes Alzheimer's. It had been thought that it was the amyloid that was causing the damage. However, several years of research and investment into drugs that prevent the accumulation of amyloid beta have ended in failure and many drug companies have abandoned Alzheimer's disease drug trials.

An alternative hypothesis suggests that amyloid is not the primary cause, but in fact, shows up because it is trying to help. One of the features of amyloid is that it has antimicrobial properties, but bacteria are not supposed to be able to get into the brain so this possibility had not previously been explored. However, new animal trials coupled with human tissue samples indicate that in fact some bacteria are able to cross the BBB and enter the brain, causing neuroinflammation and, potentially, the accumulation of amyloid beta around the site. Head to Chapter 3 to find out more on this.

The Nervous System

The nervous system is the overall name given to the nerve tissue throughout the body. It is composed of two parts:

- The Central Nervous System (CNS): the brain and the spinal cord.
- The Peripheral Nervous System (PNS): nerves connecting the CNS to the rest of the body.

The PNS can be divided again into:

- Autonomic: automatic and unconscious influence over internal organs (though it is modifiable through some conscious actions).
- Somatic: conscious control over the muscles.
- Enteric: controls activity of the gastrointestinal tract.

Of particular interest to us for the purposes of this book, because of the important influence on stress, digestion and immunity, is the subdivision of the autonomic nervous system into sympathetic and parasympathetic:

Sympathetic nervous system

You will likely be familiar with the sympathetic nervous system (SNS) by its alternative term: the 'fight or flight' response. During periods of stress or when a threat is detected, the SNS coordinates numerous physiological responses, mediated by the release and action of adrenaline, to prepare the mind and body for action.

Parasympathetic nervous system

The counterbalance to the SNS, and easily remembered as the 'rest and digest' system, the parasympathetic nervous system (PSNS) coordinates bodily activities associated with relaxation, recovery, eating, digestion and sexual activity. Since stress is one of the biggest modifiable risks to your brain health, understanding how to 'switch on' the PSNS can be helpful for looking after your mental health. Many of the tips in this book are designed to help you to do just this.

Key brain chemicals

All of your brain's functions depend on a range of endogenous (made within the body/brain) chemicals. Lifestyle factors, such as physical activity, the foods you eat and how much sleep you get, all affect the activity of these compounds. It's not essential, but you may like to know what some of these chemicals are and what they do:

Name	Function
Acetylcholine	The key compound for neuroplasticity. When an event or action is important or meaningful, acetylcholine is produced at the synapses that were activated during the event, reinforcing them and keeping them more activated. This makes acetylcholine crucial to the learning process.

Dopamine	The reward and motivation hormone. Promotes the continuation of a behaviour or activity by producing feelings of pleasure. Eating, cuddling, pictures of kittens, all upregulate dopamine secretion.
Endocannabinoids	These are chemicals synthesised within the body that can dock into cannabinoid receptors in the brain and act as signalling molecules. Their function and activity are still under investigation, but they are thought to play a role in appetite regulation, pain management, immune function, inflammation and neuronal health.
Endorphins	Endorphins are endogenous opioids that are released in response to injury, physical exertion and extreme stress (acute inflammation) to reduce pain.
Gamma-Aminobutyric acid (GABA)	This inhibitory neurotransmitter calms or slows down brain activity. Alcohol, barbiturates, benzodiazepines and theanine (a compound found in tea) all act on this system.
Glutamate	An excitatory neurotransmitter, glutamate makes it more likely that a receptor neurone will produce an action potential, and enhances synaptic plasticity, making this amino acid important for learning and memory.
Noradrenaline/norepinephrine	Prepares the brain and the body for actions. Promotes wakefulness, vigilance and attention. Crucial part of the 'fight or flight' response.

Serotonin	The good mood hormone. Serotonin is linked to good mood and feelings of well-being. It is synthesised from the essential amino acid tryptophan, which we get from food.

Takeaways

- Neurones (nerves) are the courier brain cells. They carry the messages and information between the body and the brain that are responsible for all your actions, thoughts, beliefs and ideas.
- The synapse is the location of the transmission of messages between the messenger (pre-synaptic) neurone and the receptor (post-synaptic) neurone.
- Messages are passed in the form of chemicals called neurotransmitters.
- Several types of non-neuronal cells called glia carry out important supportive functions for neurones, including providing nutrients, enhancing signalling, recycling neurotransmitters and launching an immune response.
- The blood–brain barrier is a specialised membrane that protects the brain by being highly selective about what molecules are allowed to cross over into the brain from the bloodstream.
- The areas of the brain that deal with logic and emotions are deeply interconnected. You cannot make decisions without utilising emotion networks and protecting your brain health *must* include attending to your emotions.
- Even house plants come with care instructions but we rarely think about what our brains need to be healthy. Hopefully, having a better understanding of the brain and its needs will help you to look after it. The brain is complex and requires a range of interventions to protect it. A single quick fix just won't cut it.

CHAPTER 4

The Major Players

The brain orchestrates an unfathomable range of processes and activities: from synthesising hormones and assessing incoming information for salience, to combining that new information with previous experience to come up with novel ideas. Yet, underpinning all of this activity is the basic structural and functional health of the brain. In the same way that a car that is well-maintained will last longer and be more reliable, you cannot hope to get the lasting high performance you want from your brain if it is not properly cared for and protected.

The two major players when it comes to the maintenance of brain health are the processes of *inflammation* and *neurogenesis*. The overall and continuing balance of these processes will dictate your long-term brain health.

The Immune System and Inflammation

The immune system is the body's inbuilt defence against harmful intruders such as disease-causing viruses and bacteria. Inflammation is the immune system in action, and in the majority of cases it is essential for keeping us alive. We are all familiar with the hot, painful swelling around a graze or an insect bite, or the stuffy, heavy head of a cold. This combination of redness (in fair-skinned people), swelling, heat, pain and loss of function is the visible evidence of the immune system's inflammatory response.

The immune system divides into two complementary subsystems:

1. The adaptive (specific) immune system.
2. The innate (non-specific) immune system.

The adaptive immune system is the part of our immune function that is responsive to any new or unfamiliar bacteria or viruses that we encounter. This is the system that is targeted with vaccination. A vaccine is an inert or weakened version of a disease-causing virus. When someone receives the vaccine the cells of the adaptive immune system learn through a process of trial and error what it is and how to destroy it. It is then able to manufacture more immune cells and antibodies that are specially adapted to destroy that particular virus so that, if the person is later exposed to a live version of the virus (by coming into contact with someone who is ill, for example), their body is able to quickly initiate a targeted response against it, greatly reducing the extent of the illness.

Our innate immunity is the part of our response to the pathogens that we evolved with. The bacteria and viruses that our species have come into regular contact with have shaped our immune systems so that now we are born with white blood cells with receptors on their surfaces that can recognise pathogens on first contact and launch a defence immediately. This part of the immune system is like a pair of friendly local police officers who have always worked in the same neighbourhood. After a while they get to know all the local troublemakers, the usual suspects, and as soon as they spot them (these biological criminals never reform) the officers can call in for backup to apprehend them. Under normal, healthy conditions this response is 'self-limiting', which means that after the intruders have been killed and cleaned up, the immune cells downregulate and return to a baseline level of vigilance.

But what happens if this response remains elevated for too long? Imagine our two police officers have been working for days, maybe weeks without a break. They are exhausted and in this condition they are not thinking straight. They spot what they think is a troublemaker and call for backup. However, our tired officers have made an error; maybe there isn't really anyone there or it's a case of mistaken identity. Immune activation without a real threat can lead to the body's own tissues being damaged. This is known as 'autoimmunity'. Alternatively, in a case of mistaken identity, the immune system may launch an attack on an innocent compound such as pollen or peanut protein. Allergies are a case of immune mistaken identity.

Cytokines

When the innate immune system calls for backup the signal is sent via molecules called 'cytokines'. Cytokines is the name for a group of proteins that are secreted by immune cells. Their presence alerts other cells of the immune system and the rest of the body that there is something wrong. This is really important because when the body is under threat from a virus or harmful bacteria what you want is a swift, powerful and effective response to eliminate the danger as soon as possible. When another cell receives this chemical message it can respond in a range of ways including changing its behaviours and releasing its own cytokines, to pass the message on.

Below are some examples of relevant immune actions:

- Mast cells (found in connective tissue throughout the body) secrete histamine, which causes blood vessels to dilate and makes their walls more permeable, allowing and encouraging more immune cells into the area. This accounts for much of the heat and swelling around an injury.
- Pain processes are upregulated – you become more sensitive to pain. This helps you to avoid doing further damage to the area.
- Some immune cells produce powerful chemicals, such as hydrogen peroxide, to kill pathogens and stimulate wound healing.

However, there are some circumstances in which the innate immune system is over-activated. When the immune response does not return to baseline, but remains elevated for long periods of time (weeks or months), the body is in a state of *chronic* or *systemic* inflammation. Unfortunately, all of the above processes, that are enormously helpful in an acute phase, become problematic when they are chronic:

- Excess histamine can impair healthy barrier functions (including the BBB), meaning that as well as white blood cells other cells or compounds in the blood can access the area. When cells or molecules find themselves in the wrong areas this can stimulate a further inflammatory reaction.
- You may become hypersensitive to pain so that normal bodily processes become uncomfortably painful.

- In the long-term these potent chemicals can begin to damage the body's own healthy tissues.

Chronic inflammation is implicated in a range of non-communicable (can't be passed between people) and autoimmune diseases, such as heart disease, type 2 diabetes, Alzheimer's disease, depression and gastrointestinal disorders, such as Crohn's disease and ulcerative colitis. Lifestyle factors are some of the major, modifiable contributors to chronic inflammation, meaning we each have some power to influence the direction of this process in our favour.

The Inflammation Hypothesis

The first antidepressant drugs were, as with many of our most important technologies, discovered by accident. While treating patients for tuberculosis – a serious bacterial infection – physicians observed that one of the side effects of treatment was euphoria. Patients' moods improved when they were on the treatment and, a few years later, the antibiotic iproniazid was being used to treat depression.

Iproniazid is a monoamine oxidase (MAO) inhibitor: it functions by restricting the biological action of MAO, an enzyme that degrades serotonin, dopamine and norepinephrine, neurotransmitters associated with good mood, motivation and concentration, respectively. This means that these compounds are more available at the synapse, prolonging their activity in the brain. It was also observed that suppressing tryptophan availability (tryptophan is required for serotonin production) leads to depressive symptoms.

The 'serotonin hypothesis' of depression, proposed over half a century ago, has been the dominant medical model of depression. However, as mentioned earlier, antidepressant medication does not work for all patients with depression and the rates of treatment-resistant depression continue to rise. Furthermore, even if serotonin unavailability does contribute to depression, this paradigm fails to explain *why* this happens, or how, perhaps, to restore it.

These concerns over poor response rate and the need for an explanatory model have led to a necessary reassessment of the underlying causes of depression, and psychiatric illness more generally.

Sickness behaviours

'Sickness behaviours' describes a cluster of behavioural changes that occur at the onset of physical illness or infection. They include:

- social withdrawal
- loss of interest (including in grooming and self-care)
- loss of appetite
- inactivity
- lethargy
- increased sleeping
- shivering (and raised body temperature)
- mood changes and cognitive impairments, such as difficulty making decisions

It is believed that these features evolved as part of a protective mechanism for both the individual and the tribe. Social withdrawal and loss of interest reduced the likelihood of interacting with other people and risking infecting them. Inactivity, lethargy and increased sleeping reduce energy expenditure, making more energy available for the immune response. Loss of appetite limits the availability of iron, which is essential for bacterial replication. Shivering and fever increase body temperature, which helps fight infection. Irritability and reduced self-care indicate to others that someone is unwell, stimulating innate avoidance behaviours and further reducing the risk of transmitting the infection.

Strikingly, many (if not all) of these features are part of the common symptoms of depression outlined on page 8. This observation – that people who are depressed behave in similar ways to people who are sick with a virus – contributes to the emerging evidence that depression is mediated by the immune system.

Inflammation and depression

What has the immune system got to do with the brain? The observation of the similarity between sickness behaviours and depression gave the first clue that an aspect of immune function could play a role in depression and other psychological disorders.

The medical profession has known for a long time that inflammatory illnesses also come with the risk of depression. For example, patients with psoriasis and rheumatoid arthritis, inflammatory conditions that affect the skin and joints, respectively, are more than 10 times more likely to develop depression and anxiety. Further, multiple review studies have shown that two markers of inflammation – cytokines called c-reactive protein and interleukin-6 – are consistently higher in patients with depression than non-depressed individuals. Another of these cytokines, interleukin-1α, has been shown to cause sickness behaviours. However, we cannot assume from these associations that inflammation *causes* depression – correlation is not causation. Perhaps the stress of having an uncomfortable skin condition or persistent joint pain contributes to depression independently of any inflammatory process. Or it could be that the state of becoming depressed drives the immune response. In order to test the direction of causation researchers looked at whether it was possible to promote depressive symptoms in healthy people by inducing inflammation.

To test this hypothesis, scientists created an 'immune challenge', exposing the immune system to a compound, such as a modified or inert version of a common bacterium, which will generate an inflammatory response.

In one trial, 30 people were randomly assigned to receive either an injection of modified disease-causing bacteria or a placebo (saline). The bacteria were enough to alert the immune system to launch but not active enough to cause any symptoms of illness. This is important because it means that the participants in the active arm of the trial could not tell whether they had the real substance or the placebo. It was found that the people who were injected with the modified bacteria had an elevated immune response and were significantly more depressed than those who received the placebo. Fascinatingly, the concentration of cytokines in their blood predicted the severity of depressive symptoms they reported; the higher the inflammatory response, the more depressed they were.

In another study conducted with healthy participants there was a *dose-response* effect of exposure to bacteria on mood and anxiety. This means that the higher the dose of the substance, the higher the inflammatory response and the more depressed and anxious the person felt. And a significant relationship has been demonstrated between inflammation and treatment-resistant depression, at least for some patients.

These and many other incredible studies have really transformed the scientific understanding of depression and other mood and psychiatric disorders. It suggests that, though mental health concerns have different genetic and environmental risk factors, they may share one important biological mechanism: inflammation.

How does this immune activation affect the brain? Remember that the brain is an incredibly fragile and sensitive organ, which is particularly vulnerable to inflammation. There are several important neurological processes that are interrupted by inflammation:

1. Cytokines can cause the tight junctions of the BBB to loosen, allowing cytokines, immune cells and other compounds into the brain, prompting a response from microglia, promoting further neuroinflammation.

2. High levels of circulating cytokines have been shown in animals to inhibit the process by which synapses are strengthened, a process important for learning and memory. Learning and memory deficits are common features of depression in humans.

3. Cytokines trigger a pathway that takes the essential amino acid tryptophan away from serotonin production and pushes it into the kynurenine pathway. This has a few downstream effects:
   - There is less tryptophan available for serotonin synthesis, potentially reducing serotonin availability in the brain.
   - Kynurenine is converted into kynurenic acid (KYNA) in astrocytes. KYNA upregulates the activity of dopamine receptors in the brain. This is a case of too much of a good thing because high levels of KYNA, and over-responsive dopamine receptors, are consistently identified in the brains of patients with schizophrenia. Irregularities in kynurenine

metabolism are also features of depression, Tourette's syndrome and multiple sclerosis.

- Kynurenine is converted into quinolinic acid in microglia. Quinolinic acid is powerfully neurotoxic and is associated with neurodegenerative diseases such as Alzheimer's and Parkinson's disease.

4. Cytokines also increase the reuptake of dopamine and noradrenaline in the synaptic cleft meaning these neurotransmitters are less available for normal brain functioning.

So you can see that there are many ways by which these inflammatory signalling molecules contribute to disrupted brain processes that we see in many psychiatric illnesses. This new framework may also explain *why* serotonin is often low in depressed patients. It also raises new treatment possibilities; it may soon be possible to personalise antidepressant medication by first assessing the patient's baseline cytokine levels.

As you will discover in the next chapter, stress and the stress hormones may be the final piece of the puzzle linking the known risk factors for mental illness with inflammation and the emergence of disease.

The inflammation hypothesis has shifted the way that we look at depression and other mental illnesses. Neuroinflammation, which may be triggered or exacerbated by chronic inflammation and a compromised BBB, is a key feature of neurodegenerative disorders including Alzheimer's disease, Parkinson's disease, multiple sclerosis, bipolar disorder and schizophrenia. The latest evidence indicates that lifestyle factors like nutrition (Chapter 7) and even activities like sauna use (Chapter 13) can influence these processes. This means that every day we have valuable opportunities to nudge the odds slightly more in favour of long-term brain health.

'. . . one thing is for sure: depression, and mental health problems in general, can no longer be seen only as disorders of the mind, or indeed only as disorders of the brain. The strong impact of the immune system on emotions and behaviour demonstrates that mental health is the health of the whole body.'

Professor Carmine M. Pariante, professor of biological
psychiatry at the Institute of Psychiatry, King's College, London

Neurogenesis

Neurogenesis [neuro = cell, genesis = creation] is the process of creating new brain cells and new connections between neurones in the brain. Neurogenesis is one facet of neuroplasticity, which describes the brain's capacity to remodel in response to activity and stimulus. Until recently it was believed that neurogenesis only took place during childhood and that from then on it was a downward decline as we gradually lost brain cells throughout our adult lives. However, it is now known that neurogenesis can occur in the adult brain. Research has confirmed adult neurogenesis in the hippocampus, but multipotent neurogenic precursors (cells that are able to become neurones and glia) have also been identified in the human adult amygdala and frontal cortex. This discovery has led to a plethora of new research looking at what factors contribute to neurogenesis and whether there is anything we can do to promote it.

One of the most important compounds to emerge (so far) is the protein brain-derived neurotrophic factor (BDNF, see page 28). BDNF plays several important roles in neuroplasticity:

- It promotes the growth of new neurones.
- It helps new cells to survive.
- It supports the survival of pre-existing neurones.
- It supports the development of synapses – the communication junctions between brain cells.

Neurogenesis is crucial to the process of learning and memory. When you learn something new, whether it is a fact about the brain or how to ride a bike, the brain has to accommodate this new information. This may require new brain cells or new connections between existing ones. This means that every time you learn something you are building and shaping your brain. This building and reshaping process underlies one of the most important brain-health concepts in this book: 'cognitive reserve'.

Cognitive reserve
Whether you have started paying into one or not, most people agree that having a pension plan is a good idea. The premise of a pension is pretty simple: while you are working you pay in small amounts of money that accumulate to a significant amount for you to draw on when you retire. Having a nest egg like this also means that, if there is an emergency, you have a safety net to fall back on. You can think of the principle of cognitive reserve as a pension plan for your brain.

The term cognitive reserve was coined in a research paper published in 1988 to describe some surprising post-mortem findings. Typically, in Alzheimer's disease, there is a high degree of correlation between the level of memory and functional impairment a person displays when they are alive and the amount of damage visible in their brains after they die. That is to say, the more severe a person's memory problems the more brain lesions they have. However, this study of 137 elderly residents of a New York nursing home showed something remarkable. There was a subgroup of residents who, when tested on their memory, scored the same as healthy older people, that is, they showed no signs of Alzheimer's disease. Yet, when their brains were assessed after their deaths, they actually had *more* physical damage to their brains than many of those who had received a diagnosis of dementia. Somehow, despite having the physical signs of advanced brain disease, this group of patients had escaped showing symptoms while they were alive. It is like someone feeling no pain and walking normally on a broken ankle. How could this be?

The researchers noticed one important feature of the brains of this group of residents: they were heavier than the others. They surmised that this special group of residents had started out with bigger, heavier brains before they developed dementia. To put it another way, this special group of residents had more stored up in their brain pensions than the others. This meant that when dementia started to take cells away they still had more than enough left over to function normally.

But this raises an important question: were they just lucky? Perhaps this group were just born with bigger brains. Or was there something about their lives that helped to build extra brain reserve? Further research seemed to provide an answer. For example, it has been consistently found that a person's level of education influences their risk of developing dementia and Alzheimer's disease. The more years of formal education you have (i.e. the more years of learning you accumulate), the lower your risk of dementia. This result seems to hold in spite of other factors such as health and socio-economic status. The reviews and meta-analyses that have been conducted so far show support for the cognitive reserve hypothesis. This is a powerful finding: it means that, starting right now, we have the opportunity to start building that brain pension plan. And the earlier you start, the better.

The information in this book is designed to help you to understand what aspects of your current lifestyle might be contributing to inflammation or downregulated neurogenesis (so that you can do less of these activities). It also describes what lifestyle habits are associated with increased levels of neurogenesis so that you can start building your brain pension plan.

Takeaways

- Inflammation is immune activation. In the short-term, inflammation protects us from harmful bugs, but chronic inflammation is associated with serious physical and psychological illness.
- Cytokines are signalling proteins released by immune cells in response to an immunological challenge.
- Immunological inflammation within the body may be a crucial biological mechanism underlying depression and other unhealthy mental states.
- Cytokines can inhibit the release of key neurotransmitters such as serotonin, dopamine and noradrenaline.
- Cytokines increase the reuptake of serotonin in the brain, meaning that less serotonin is available at the synapse (e.g. this is the opposite of what antidepressant medication is designed to do).
- Cytokines interfere with tryptophan metabolism, meaning that less of this essential amino acid is available for serotonin synthesis.
- Understanding what is contributing to elevated inflammation may help to improve treatment and outcomes for patients.

- Neurogenesis is the process of creating new neurones and connections in the brain.
- Cognitive reserve, the principle of building up extra brain volume, is like a pension plan for the brain. Current research suggests that BDNF is a key factor in this process. Throughout this book there is information on the lifestyle factors that have been shown to increase levels of this important compound.

CHAPTER 5

How Stress Affects
Brain and Mental Health

Many people will be familiar with the experience of psychological pressure that accompanies a looming deadline or a demanding activity like public speaking. To a degree this pressure can be positive; it helps you to focus your attention on the task at hand and sometimes the adrenaline of an acutely stressful event can improve performance. However, pressure becomes stress when we begin to feel that the demands upon us are outstripping or eroding our ability to cope, and the things that create stress may vary within individuals (depending on what else is going on) and between individuals (depending on personal resilience factors). So, we might normally be able to cope with work pressure but feel unable to cope if we are also dealing with a relationship break-up at the same time. Similarly, the stress that one person can tolerate might be overwhelming stress for another. This means that stress and stress management is not simply a set of rules that need to be followed, but a negotiation between the pressures, the resilience factors, and the available coping mechanisms.

The Anatomy of Stress

Stress may be psychological (e.g. work deadlines), chemical (e.g. smoking) and physiological (e.g. illness), but it is always biological. That is to say, whatever the source of stress, it creates measurable changes in the body. I want to emphasise this because people tend to be very dismissive of the real effects of emotional stress both on their mental and physical health. Simply because they cannot *see* the effects, they discredit and judge themselves for failing to cope or being 'weak'. However, the perceived separation between mind and body is both arbitrary and false, and, as you will see, the biological processes are real, as are the physical effects and, no matter the source, stress should be taken seriously.

The stress response is an evolutionary mechanism that is mediated by the sympathetic nervous system (SNS) and developed to protect the body at times of short-lived risk.

Let's imagine you are taking a peaceful walk through a field on a sunny day. You feel calm, you are breathing gently and your gaze is soft, not focused on anything in particular but taking in a panoramic view of everything around you. Then, out of the corner of your eye, you spot something that seems out of place in this scene, a sudden movement, the shadow of a shape. Immediately your eyes shift from gentle panoramic vision to sharp focus as your brain tries to identify what that shape is. This information is transmitted to the amygdala, the threat detection centre, which plays the crucial role of adding meaning to what you have seen. Is it dangerous or benign? This decision will be based partly on previous experience and partly on in-built instinctive reactions. For example, falling objects will almost always provoke a startle response even when it's just a leaf falling from a tree.* But this isn't a falling leaf, and if the amygdala recognises a threat it will send a signal to the hypothalamus, which subsequently signals to the adrenal glands. This pair of glands, which sit on top of the kidneys, releases adrenaline into the bloodstream, which, along with cortisol, initiates a raft of physiological processes in your body:

Action	Function	Chronic secondary effects
Heart beats faster, blood vessels constrict, blood moved out of the gastrointestinal tract to the limbs.	Blood available to the arms and legs in order to be ready to fight, defend or run.	Elevated blood pressure puts stress on the heart. Digestion halted or significantly impaired; gastrointestinal symptoms.
Bronchioles dilate.	Breathing rate increases. Lung capacity increases to supply muscles and brain with necessary oxygen for increased activity and alertness.	Can promote chronic inflammation of the airway. May worsen symptoms of asthma and other lung problems.

* Horror movies exploit our innate startle response with jump-scares – those moments, where after a build-up of tension, a character or loud noise will appear out of nowhere.

Glucose and triglycerides (fats) released into the blood.	Emergency energy available for action.	Long-term elevated blood sugar contributes to raised insulin levels that may precipitate insulin insensitivity and prediabetes.
Cortisol suppresses the action of insulin, the hormone that promotes the storage of glucose.		Fats that remain in the bloodstream are more likely to be oxidised, a process that contributes to atherosclerosis (clogged arteries).
		May contribute to weight gain and the accumulation of visceral fat (around the organs), which is a risk factor for heart disease.
Healthy immune function suppressed.	Immune function has a high energetic demand so this saves energy for other immediate use.	Increased susceptibility to illness.
Increased attention to potential risks in the environment.	Promotes readiness to act.	Long-term attention to negative stimuli is a behavioural risk for depression.

You can see how, in acute situations, this set of automatic responses to stress is effective for managing threats. Yet, if sustained, the same responses can contribute to a number of negative physical and psychological states. In addition, it has been established that chronically elevated cortisol increases the risk for many illnesses.

Chronic Stress

Chronic stress is perhaps the single biggest risk to brain health. Elevated levels of stress hormones cause dendrites (see page 27) to shrink and cell bodies to die. The hippocampus is rich in receptors for stress hormones but in excess these stress hormones can cause damage. Animal models have shown that prolonged stress suppresses neurogenesis in the hippocampus, the organ that plays such an important role in memory and where we want to be upregulating the production of new connections. Further, activity is suppressed in the prefrontal cortex (PFC), important for executive processes such as decision-making, planning and reason, while there is more activity in the amygdala, the brain's threat detection centre.

Chronic stress is a known risk factor for Alzheimer's. In the brains of mice engineered to be vulnerable to Alzheimer's-like disease, chronically elevated stress hormones worsen the illness. These animal observations also translate to humans. When a group of healthy older adults was assessed over a period of seven years, those with chronic and high levels of stress hormones had smaller hippocampi and worse memory performance than those with moderate levels. Another group of researchers assessed healthy older adults, all aged over 70 and none of whom had signs of mild cognitive impairment (MCI), a common precursor to dementia. They were followed up about four years later and those who reported higher levels of stress had a 30 per cent increased risk of cognitive decline than those who were less stressed.

Chronic stress and inflammation

Chronic stress also drives neuroinflammation. It is well established from animal models that chronic stress activates microglia. Under a range of stressful conditions inflammatory activity can be seen in the hippocampus, the PFC and the amygdala, areas with high numbers of cortisol receptors. Increased microglial activation has been identified in the brains of human patients with diagnoses of anxiety, depression and schizophrenia, as well as Alzheimer's disease.

Strikingly, early life stress seems to prime microglia, lowering the threshold for later activation. This would suggest that people who experience difficult or traumatic experiences early in life would be at higher risk of psychological illness and, indeed, adverse childhood experiences are associated with greater incidence of mental illness.

Physical symptoms

People often think about stress as a solely psychological experience but, as we have discussed, stress is biological and the stress hormones influence almost every system in the body, from brain cells to blood sugar. As such, the effects of chronic stress are revealed in many physical symptoms. Many of the physical symptoms people present with at the GP are thought to be driven by stress. It is worth being familiar with some of the bodily manifestations of chronic stress so that you can assess and address them as early as possible:

- headache, migraine
- back pain
- heart palpitations, chest pain
- breathlessness
- digestive problems
- significant weight change
- sexual dysfunction, erectile dysfunction, loss of libido
- excessive use of stimulants and substances: caffeine, cocaine, alcohol
- poor sleep – taking longer to fall asleep, frequent waking, waking not feeling refreshed

Irritable bowel syndrome

Irritable bowel syndrome (IBS) is a common disorder that affects between 15 and 20 per cent of Western populations. The disorder is characterised by uncomfortable and sometimes embarrassing gut symptoms – such as bloating, cramping, wind, abdominal pain, constipation or diarrhoea, or a combination of these – that can seriously impair the sufferer's quality of life.

IBS is a functional disorder of the gut. This means that in IBS there is an impairment of the normal healthy functioning of the gut, in the absence of the presence of a disease. If a doctor were to investigate the gut with an endoscope there would be no signs of polyps, obstruction or illness. It is also a diagnosis of exclusion; in order to make a diagnosis of IBS, a doctor will first have to eliminate the possibility that the symptoms might be caused by an organic disease.

Perhaps understandably, particularly with an abundance of conflicting information available about food and nutrition, when people begin to experience these symptoms, they will often presume it is their diet causing the problem, perhaps changing their diet or cutting out a food group to try to fix it. However, this can often do more harm than good, because radical dietary changes can (further) disturb the composition of the gut microbiome, which can exacerbate symptoms.

What is often ignored is that IBS is a stress-sensitive disorder. Not only can stress trigger flare-ups in symptoms, but the interaction of stress, inflammation and the gut–brain axis can perpetuate the disorder. This is demonstrated in research that shows that psychotherapy and yoga are as effective as dietary changes for managing IBS.

If you think you might be suffering from IBS, please see your GP or a specialist dietitian before making any dietary changes.

Psychological symptoms

In addition, here are the often overlooked psychological signs that you might be under excess pressure:

- increased aggression, short temper or frustration
- anxiety
- low mood or depression
- apathy, loss of interest
- overwhelm
- poor concentration or forgetfulness
- procrastination or lack of motivation
- cynicism
- loss of confidence/self-esteem
- impaired memory function
- impaired emotional responses
- social withdrawal

Left untreated, chronic stress can lay the biophysiological foundations for depression and other mental illnesses. This is why it is so important to take stress seriously, to do what you can to reduce sources of stress in your life and to ensure that periods of stress are followed by adequate recovery.

Are You Burned Out?

'Burnout' is the term given to the persistent experience of physical and psychological exhaustion associated with long-term work stress, though it is common for people who are carers for relatives to also experience burnout. We may all experience very intense or stressful days at work, but in ideal circumstances they are a rarity and we recover quickly after a good night of rest and relaxation. When it comes to burnout there is often little opportunity for proper recovery. Instead, the pressures of the job feel overwhelming and relentless and we have insufficient time to recuperate. At best, this can leave you feeling as though you are 'running on fumes'; never really fully yourself. At worst, you can feel always on the brink of tears, while conversely cut off from emotional connection with your friends and family, with little time, interest or energy for personal interests. Burnout is also linked to an increased risk of depression.

The following factors are associated with the risk of experiencing burnout:

- excessive workload
- lack of control, autonomy or decision authority
- insufficient reward
- lack of peer support/difficult workplace relationships
- lack of fairness
- conflict of values
- job insecurity

The following scale will give an indication of how burned out you may be. If you feel you might be suffering from burnout, it is important to try to address this as soon as possible. Which of the factors listed above do you think are most relevant to your situation? Is it possible to speak to your boss or the HR department to try to address them? Working with a therapist might help you to identify the particular areas of difficulty and help you to develop strategies for raising or resolving the issues.

	A	B	C	D	E
Definition	Never/Almost never	Rarely	Sometimes	Often	Always
Value	0	25	50	75	100

Work-related Burnout

Do you feel worn out at the end of the working day?	A	B	C	D	E
Are you exhausted in the morning at the thought of another day at work?	A	B	C	D	E
Do you feel that every working hour is tiring for you?	A	B	C	D	E
Is your work emotionally exhausting?	A	B	C	D	E
Does your work frustrate you?	A	B	C	D	E
Do you feel burnt out because of your work?	A	B	C	D	E

Answer each of the questions as honestly as possible. Add up your scores and then divide the final number by 6. Scores of 0–49 are 'low', 50–74 are considered 'moderate', 75–99 are high, and a score of 100 is considered severe burnout.

Adapted from the Copenhagen Burnout Scale.

Not All Stress Is Created Equal

We have established that the body has evolved adaptive mechanisms to manage occasional, acute stress, and we have seen how, if the stressor persists, these usually adaptive mechanisms can become maladaptive and contribute to disease processes in the body. But that is not the end of the story when it comes to stress. There is another type of stress that we should all be exposing ourselves to more often in the pursuit of healthy brains: 'hormesis', the good stress.

Hormesis may be physiological or psychological in nature. Exercise is a good example – when you lift weights, you apply a short-term, manageable pressure to the muscle. The body responds to this stress by upregulating muscular repair processes and making the muscles more able to tolerate the same amount of stress post-recovery i.e. becoming stronger. We see this adaptive hormesis in action all over the body. In fact, many of the recommendations in this book, such as exercise and heat exposure, rely on taking advantage of hormesis in different ways.

The stress equation

One way of looking at health is as a relative balance of stress, hormesis and recovery:

$$\frac{Stress}{Hormesis + Recovery} = Health$$

Too much stress and/or too little hormesis and recovery will lead to poorer outcomes. Conversely, frequent hormetic stress and recovery build resilience to negative and chronic stress.

Takeaways

- Stress is an experience associated with tension, nervousness or strain. It may have physical, environmental or psychological triggers, but all have measurable biological effects on the body.
- Stress falls into three categories: acute, chronic and hormesis.
- We evolved a stress response to allow us to adapt and respond to short-term environmental stressors. Unfortunately, our modern lives provide many sources of long-term or chronic stress.
- Chronic stress activates inflammation in the body and the brain.
- Regular exposure to hormesis, with sufficient recovery, is associated with better health and greater resilience.

Now you know the basics about the brain, the major players of brain health (inflammation and neurogenesis) and how different types of stress affect brain and mental health, we are ready to get to grips with how different lifestyle habits influence these factors and how you can create your own brain-healthy lifestyle.

CHAPTER 6

The Importance of Sleep

The last few years have seen a welcome rise in interest around the importance of sleep. This renaissance in attention to sleep is long overdue and it's about much more than just feeling a little more refreshed. The journey to a more resilient brain and improved mental health starts in bed.

I worked for a few years in a corporate law firm in the heart of London. The firm managed mergers and acquisitions between global businesses and banks and, of course, it was expected that the highly paid solicitors working on the files would be constantly available for their clients, who might be located anywhere in the world, in any time zone. In these sorts of working environments, it does not matter that it's 3am; the expectation is that the lawyers make themselves available to respond to the client's needs. When it comes to closing a deal or preparing for court, this mentality goes into overdrive. It is not uncommon for associates to have their holidays cancelled and to be expected to stay up all night in order to work on a case.

At that time I was a trainee psychologist and I watched with great interest (and occasional horror) at what are in fact very typical working conditions in law, finance, advertising, media and, of course, healthcare. In my humble opinion, this lack of sleep, which is just considered part of the job, was wreaking havoc on the lawyers' emotional well-being.

There is a great deal of evidence now to support the observation that inadequate sleep was negatively impacting not only the lawyers' emotions but also their broader brain function and mental health. To better understand the relationship between sleep and mental health we need to appreciate the structure and function of sleep.

Circadian Rhythmicity

We evolved in environments devoid of artificial light, and so our physiological patterns of activity and rest correspond to the evolutionary light availability; that is, we are driven to be more active during daylight hours and to rest and sleep during darkness. But it is not just wakefulness and sleep that are governed by this daylight/darkness pattern; metabolism, the gut microbiome and even wound healing all follow this cyclical course.

Your brain and body work best when you stick to this pattern of daylight activity and night-time sleep. However, modern urban life provides us with lots of reasons to stay up late and innumerable sources of artificial light: from overhead bulbs and street lamps to supermarket lighting and handheld devices.

The majority of the cells in your body have their own chemical timekeeper, but the 'master clock' that coordinates the overall bodily rhythm, called the 'suprachiasmatic nuclei' (SCN), sits deep in the brain in the hypothalamus. Specialised cells in the retina convey information about external light levels and transmit this directly to the SCN, which adjusts its own pattern accordingly. Information about ambient light levels is then transmitted to the pineal gland, which secretes a hormone called melatonin. Melatonin, which peaks during darkness hours, is the body's sleep-promotor, kick-starting the physiological changes that prepare the body for sleep.

Sleep Architecture

During sleep your brain cycles through different stages, which can be measured by monitoring the pattern of electrical signals made by neurones:

These varying stages of sleep correspond to different but equally important brain functions.

Light sleep: stages 1 and 2
These first stages of sleep are considered induction and transition stages from which you can be easily woken.

Deep sleep: stages 3 (and 4)
Until recently, these stages were considered separate but it is now common to view them as one single stage of slow wave sleep. This is the stage of sleep from which it is most difficult to be woken.

Slow wave sleep is crucial for the process of memory consolidation, when information from the day is relocated from the short-term storage area of the hippocampus to long-term storage elsewhere in the brain. Synapses are also augmented, priming them for later activation (learning). So sleep both prepares the brain to learn new things and helps to ensure that new information is retained in the long-term.

Sleep stages

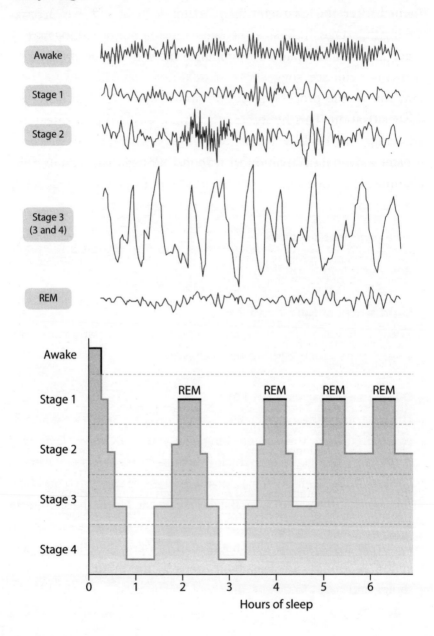

THE IMPORTANCE OF SLEEP

Rapid eye movement (REM) sleep

Named after the characteristic darting pattern the eyes make during this stage, REM sleep is where most of our dreaming takes place and is accompanied by reduced activity in the amygdala. Growing evidence suggests that dreaming may play an important role in the processing of emotional memories and distress desensitisation. This hypothesis is supported by recent research showing that healthy people who are sleep-deprived express greater amygdala activation in response to negative stimuli, for example.

The glymphatic system

The lymphatic system is part of the body's fluid circulation and is comprised of vessels that collect the fluid (lymph) that gets pushed out of the blood vessels during normal circulation. Lymphatic vessels return the lymph back into the bloodstream, helping to maintain the fluid balance between blood and the body's tissues.

One of the most profound advances in our understanding of the functions and importance of sleep came from the discovery of the glymphatic system, the brain's version of the lymphatic system. During sleep synapses expand by up to 60 per cent (mouse model) and cerebral spinal fluid flushes in and clears the brain of toxic metabolites and proteins such as amyloid beta. In fact, clearance of amyloid during sleep is twice that seen during waking.

The Impact of Sleep on Brain Health

When it comes to protecting your brain and your long-term mental health there is probably no more comprehensive intervention than sleep, and the relationship between sleep and mental illness has been observed for many years. Sleep disturbance is seen in a range of psychiatric disorders including:

- depression
- anxiety disorders such as generalised anxiety disorder, panic disorder and post-traumatic stress disorder
- ADHD
- bipolar disorder
- eating disorders
- dementia and Alzheimer's disease

For a long time it was believed that poor sleep was simply a symptom of these psychiatric illnesses. However, it is now known that sleep disturbance is a contributing factor in the development and maintenance of these illnesses.

Depression

Up to 84 per cent of depressed people also report poor sleep, and sleep issues often precede mood changes in depression. There are also associated changes in sleep architecture, with depressed people taking longer to fall asleep, waking more often during the night and experiencing a higher proportion of REM sleep than non-depressed individuals. This means that these brains are not getting enough of the non-REM sleep during which memories are consolidated and the brain is cleared of the build-up of potentially harmful waste products.

Anxiety

People with insomnia are over 17 times more likely to have troubling levels of anxiety than average sleepers. Research indicates that when the quality of sleep goes down, the level of anxiety goes up. Additionally, therapeutic interventions designed to treat insomnia and improve sleep quality are also effective at reducing anxiety symptoms, presenting a valuable treatment opportunity for some of the up to 30 per cent of people who will be troubled by anxiety during their lifetime.

Alzheimer's disease

One of the most profound associations between sleep and brain health is seen in dementia, where there is a substantial overlap between sleep disorders and cognitive decline. Even brief bouts of poor sleep reduce the brain's ability to clear amyloid beta, and mid-life insomnia is associated with an increased risk of Alzheimer's disease. Consistently, a history of poor sleep increases a person's risk of developing cognitive impairment and Alzheimer's. Sadly, the relationship between sleep impairments and dementia may be circular – poor sleep degrades brain health leading to a brain that struggles to generate healthy sleep.

Immunity

Another striking effect of sleep disturbance is how much and how quickly it affects the immune system. Just one night of poor sleep can disrupt immunity, making you more susceptible to viruses. A small trial set out to simulate the average sleep habits during a normal working week reported that sleep deprivation altered the function of 117 different genes, many of them linked to regulation of the immune system. While some of these changes disappeared after sleep was restored, some of the effects persisted and, long-term, could contribute to chronic inflammation. But even short bursts of sleep deprivation can impair our immune function, with one trial showing that after just two days of insufficient sleep circulating levels of natural killer (NK) cells were significantly reduced. NK cells are part of the innate immune system and are the first line of defence against virally-infected and cancerous cells.

Activity and exposure to light during the evening suppresses melatonin production, which as well as promoting sleep plays a communication function with the immune system. Cells of the innate immune system have receptors for melatonin and the hormone can modulate immune function. The mechanics are still being unveiled in pre-clinical research, but melatonin signalling may influence autoimmunity, inflammation and some forms of cancer. For example, night shift work forces the body out of circadian alignment; the body is compelled to be active during genetically encoded periods of rest, repair and inactivity. This action of sleep deprivation on immunity is one of the reasons that working night shifts was listed in 2007 as a probable carcinogen by the World Health Organization.

Medication and Sleep

Sleep deprivation is a form of torture. Whether you have a new baby, inconsiderate neighbours or simply live on a busy road, the distress caused by being unable to sleep is real. For this reason I undertook additional training in sleep assessment and include a sleep diary as part of the standard clinical assessment for new patients. If someone comes to therapy and reports poor sleep as a symptom, addressing this issue moves up the list of clinical priorities. Quite simply, you will not get very far in your treatment if you can't sleep: your memory consolidation will be impaired as will your brain's capacity to form new connections, which is one of the principle functions of therapy. So, before we even attempt to tackle the psychological issues that bring patients to my consultation room, helping them to sleep is one of our most important tasks.

Sedation is not sleep

I am not against psychiatric medication in principle, and have worked with many people who have found antidepressant medication to be an invaluable part of their treatment and recovery. However, there are a number of known negative consequences that these pharmaceuticals have on sleep:

Medication	Known effects on sleep
Amitriptyline (Elavil and Vanatrip)	REM sleep suppression Increased stage 2 sleep
Citalopram (Celexa or Cipramil)	Insomnia REM suppression Increased eye movements in non-REM sleep
Dapoxetine (Priligy)	Insomnia
Escitalopram (Cipralex or Lexapro)	Insomnia REM suppression Increased eye movements in non-REM sleep
Fluoxetine (Oxactin and Prozac)	Insomnia
Fluvoxamine (Faverin)	Insomnia

Mirtazapine (Remeron)	Sedation REM sleep suppression
Paroxetine (Paxil or Seroxat)	Insomnia REM suppression Increased eye movements in non-REM sleep
Sertraline (Lustral or Zoloft)	Insomnia REM suppression Increased eye movements in non-REM sleep
Venlafaxine (Effexor)	Insomnia REM suppression Increased eye movements in non-REM sleep
Vortioxetine (Viibryd)	Night sweats

In addition, despite the name, sleeping pills typically provide sedation rather than promoting true sleep.

There is a dilemma here: on the one hand it is incredibly important that people who are suffering from depression and sleep disturbance find some relief; on the other, if we are wanting to optimise brain health and recovery it may be that these drugs actually interfere with one of the most restorative processes available to us – proper natural sleep.

The value of restoring true sleep over medication-induced sedation has now been medically recognised. In 2016 the American College of Physicians published new guidelines recommending that sleeping pills should not be the first-line treatment for sleep disturbance. Similarly, the National Institute for Health and Care Excellence, which sets guidelines for healthcare professionals in the UK, recommends that patients should be offered cognitive behavioural therapy for insomnia (CBT-I) in the first instance (see page 83). This evidence-based and effective form of talking therapy involves:

- Educating patients about sleep hygiene.
- Introducing healthy sleep-promoting behaviours.
- Helping to manage negative and anxious thoughts about sleep, reducing 'sleep worry'.

Both online and in-person versions of CBT-I have been shown to be safe, reduce sleep latency (how long it takes to fall asleep), improve sleep quality and daily functioning.

Again, I am not suggesting that people should not be prescribed medication, and there should be no shame at all in taking a prescribed drug to support you with your mental health. Please do not make any changes to your prescribed medication without the consultation and agreement of your prescribing physician. My concern is with the potential negative unintended consequences that medication might have on other aspects of a person's sleep and it is something that both patients and practitioners should be aware of.

Sleep inertia
Ever wake up feeling a bit dazed and confused? A bit foggy-headed even when you have had a decent night's sleep? This is usually the point at which many people reach for a cup of coffee to 'wake them up' and, while caffeine can temporarily increase alertness, it may not be the caffeine that is doing all the work.

Sleep inertia (SI) is the term given to the period between waking up and full wakefulness when you feel a bit drowsy and clumsy. During SI your brain is transitioning between the processes that occur during sleep to those required for waking function and it takes about 15–30 minutes depending on how much sleep you have had, the phase of sleep you were in when you woke up and how much sleep debt you have accumulated.

The crucial thing to know about SI is that, during this period, a broad range of cognitive functions are significantly impaired: memory, reaction time, logical reasoning, decision-making, risk assessment and coordination have all been shown to be much worse during SI.

What this means in practice is that you should avoid any activity that requires high levels of attention or risk in the first 30 minutes after waking. The most obvious risk is driving. Whether you're a parent jumping in the car for the school run or a lorry driver waking up after a nap you will need to allow time for your brain function to return to normal waking levels to avoid the risk of drowsy driving.

Finding Your Rhythm

On top of the circadian rhythm, there are a number of shorter (ultradian) cycles that repeat throughout the day. One of these, the basic rest–activity cycle (BRAC), is thought to be roughly 90 minutes long and is identifiable as oscillations between alertness and sleepiness. It may vary between 80 and 120 minutes between individuals, but it is stable for each person i.e. if yours is 85 minutes long it will be stable at that rhythm while your partner might be a stable 100-minute cycler.

The image below shows a 90-minute cycle. At the peak of the wave you will feel at your most alert. This would be a good time to tackle any particularly demanding tasks. At the trough you will feel tired and perhaps a bit daydreamy. This might be a good time to take a break or work on more abstract, creative activities.

BRAC – Basic Rest-Activity Cycle

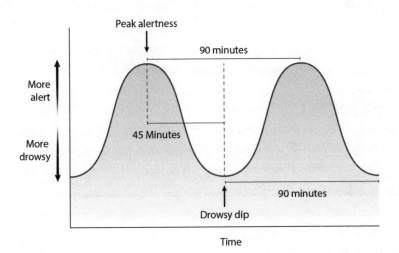

You can try to find your own pattern by looking out for moments in your day when you experience dips in alertness i.e. when you yawn. Simply take a piece of paper and place it somewhere handy (on your desk or in your pocket). Then, assuming you have had a good night's sleep and are not excessively tired, track the times across the day when you yawn. Do this for three days and take an average.

Day 1	Interval
10am	
11.37am	97
1.15pm	98
2.25pm	70
4.04pm	99
5.45pm	101
7.11pm	86
8.39pm	88
9.53pm	74
11.32pm	99
Average	90

In the above example my BRAC is about 90 minutes long. I can use this information to identify when would be the best time for me to go to bed. For example, it would not make sense for me to try to go to sleep at 9pm because I would be shifting into a peak of alertness so I am likely to find it very difficult to drift off. I should aim to be in bed for 10pm or 11.30pm to get the best chances of catching the dip in alertness.

Maybe you have read online or in health magazines all about sleep hygiene and the importance of a routine and have been valiantly trying to go to bed at a set time, yet struggle to get off to sleep, lying there for half an hour or more before you can drift off. It may be that you are trying to go to sleep against your own rhythm. There is a BRAC Tracker on page 313 so that you can try out this method and see if it helps.

Morning larks vs night owls

A search on social media for #5amClub returns hundreds of thousands of posts outlining the benefits of waking at this hour. An early start is culturally associated with ambition, motivation, hard work and success. Moreover, Western society is organised around the morning, with schools usually starting at around 8.45am in the UK and work at around 9am, meaning that students and workers wake up just after 7am on average, often earlier. As a consequence, people who habitually wake later in the day or struggle with early starts tend to be perceived negatively, as lazy or disorganised. Even demonstrably 'Type A' (competitive and goal-driven) clients will criticise their own inability to feel good and be productive in the morning.

There is, however, some solace for people who struggle to leap out of bed in the early hours; they may simply be 'night owls' rather than 'morning larks', and this tendency is genetically determined – it is just how you are made. Our peak times for physical and mental performance are influenced by our relative morningness or eveningness. For example, forcing a night owl to wake early every morning means they will be getting less good-quality sleep than if they woke later in the morning, with the negative effects on brain health associated with that. Where possible, it is therefore advisable to try to organise your daily activities around your personal 'chronotype' to maximise your opportunity for good-quality sleep.

Don't know your chronotype? You can find an online version of the 'Morningness-Eveningness Questionnaire' at: www.cet-surveys.com

Sleep-tracking devices

In the field of sleep management there is growing awareness of what has been dubbed 'orthosomnia', driven by the rise in sleep tracking apps and devices. Sleep trackers are wearable devices (often in the style of a watch or a ring) that record bodily movements during sleep and transmit the data to a smartphone app that generates a report that claims to be an accurate record of sleep duration and quality. However, sleep professionals do not generally endorse the data derived from commercial trackers as they tend to not correlate to measures used in formal clinical sleep assessments. A group of researchers led by clinical psychologist Dr Kelly Glazer Baron, at the University of Utah, worry that, at least for some people, the information they get from their sleep-tracking devices might be doing more harm than good:

> Despite multiple validation studies that have demonstrated consumer-wearable sleep tracking devices are unable to accurately discriminate stages of sleep and have poor accuracy in detecting wake after sleep onset, we found patients' perceptions difficult to alter. In addition, lack of transparency in the device algorithms makes it impossible to know how accurate they are even under the best circumstances.

A series of case reports published in the *Journal of Clinical Sleep Medicine* described how, for some patients, the use of trackers 'reinforce sleep-related anxiety or perfectionism'. Since a significant proportion of sleep problems are attributable to dysfunctional beliefs about sleep, there may be a subgroup of patients for whom the use of trackers is actually exacerbating their sleep problems.

This is an example of the risk of the extremes. There is no such thing as the perfect night's sleep or a perfect sleeper. For most people the issue is simply trying to ensure that they get *enough*. Insufficient sleep rather than 'imperfect' sleep is the main concern for most people.

How to Deal with Sleep Problems

There is no shortage of information available online for what is termed 'sleep hygiene' – activities designed to help improve your sleep. However, there has been some criticism that the current sleep hygiene recommendations have been drawn from the unnatural environments of sleep research laboratories, so they may not be directly applicable to everyday life. For example, some studies testing the effect of caffeine on sleep gave participants the equivalent of six cups of coffee just before bed! Clearly not a great idea, but what about smaller doses of caffeine earlier in the day? As with all research outcomes, recommendations need to be tailored to the individual. What follows is general advice drawn from the extant research literature for treating insomnia. You are advised to adapt these recommendations to suit your needs and lifestyle.

Sleep psychologist and Clinical Director of Sleep Unlimited, Dr David Lee, developed the R.E.S.T. programme, a CBT-I protocol based on what are currently understood to be the most effective elements of CBT-I. R.E.S.T. is an acronym for the stages of the treatment:

1. **R**outine
2. **E**nvironment

3. Stimulation Control
4. Thinking

Routine

Sleep likes routine, and that routine should be specific to you, accommodating factors such as your chronotype and whether you are a long (8–9 hours) or short (6–7 hours) sleeper.

- Take the Morningness-Eveningness Questionnaire (page 81) and find out your chronotype. Do what you can to organise your activities and your bedtime routine around your natural sleep/wake schedule.
- Try not to spend too long in bed either side of your actual sleep requirement. For example, don't get into bed at 8pm if you don't intend to fall asleep until 9.30pm. Similarly, when you wake up try not to hang around in bed too long before getting up and starting your day.
- If you have been in bed for 15–20 minutes and cannot drift off, 'get up, get out'. Get out of bed, go to another room and do something non-stimulating (no horror movies, alcohol, nicotine or caffeine). Try some easy reading, journaling, meditation or a breath practice until you feel sleepy again, then return to bed and try again.
- Maintain your sleep routine throughout the week, including weekends.

Environment

Make the bedroom environment conducive to good sleep:

- Make sure your bed is as comfortable as possible. Choose a mattress softness or hardness that suits you. The same goes for pillows.

- A cool room (around 20°C) is generally recommended, but there may be individual differences here. In addition, a woman's body temperature changes during her menstrual cycle, which may affect what external temperature feels comfortable. Don't let your feet get too cold: it can cause blood to be redirected to the trunk and keep body temperature elevated, which may interfere with sleep.
- Light is a powerful stimulator for the brain and circadian rhythmicity. Try to block out as much light as possible. Invest in thick curtains or blackout blinds. An eye mask is a good option if new curtains are not affordable. If you have dimmer switches fitted in your home turn down your household lights at least an hour before bed.
- Noise can be both an interruption and a distraction. Unfortunately, there is often not much we can do about it, especially if you live near a main road or airport, or live in a home with thin walls and noisy neighbours. If possible, locate the bedroom in the quietest spot in your home and use ear plugs if you need to.
- Tidy up. For some people clutter and mess can increase levels of arousal/stress (others don't mind so much). Keeping the bedroom clear can induce a sense of calm, which can promote sleep.
- No work in the bedroom. Aim to keep the bedroom as a place for sleep and sex only; watch TV, scroll social media, read, eat and work somewhere else. This helps to create a psychological association of the bedroom as a place to sleep.

Could a weighted blanket help?

Researchers working with children with a diagnosis of autism found that applying physical pressure (via rollers and Swiss balls for example) was effective at reducing stress and anxiety. A similar effect has been demonstrated in adults. (I myself find it difficult to sleep without a blanket over me, even during the summer months.)

These observations have led to the development of weighted blankets: otherwise normal blankets lined with metal chain, plastic pellets or glass beads to create additional pressure. A small clinical trial published in 2015 found that people with insomnia who slept with a weighted blanket (most chose 8kg blankets) fell asleep faster, slept longer and moved less during their sleep. The participants also reported feeling more refreshed on waking after sleep under the weighted blanket.

More research is required on larger groups of people to give a clearer sense of the efficacy of weighted blankets in supporting sleep quality or ameliorating insomnia. However, this non-pharmacological intervention might be worth trying for those with sleep issues who are able to afford it. Give it a go for four weeks.

Stimulation control

Stimulation is the enemy of sleep. Some substances and habits heighten physiological and psychological arousal and, if you have trouble sleeping, eliminating them can help improve sleep quality.

• Try not to go to bed on a full stomach. Digestion raises body temperature, impairing sleep onset, and any sugars in your meal will be absorbed quickly, making you feel more alert.

- Avoid drinking too much liquid before bed. Getting up several times in the night to pee is a major cause of sleep fragmentation. Keep a bottle of water by the bed so you can rehydrate in the morning instead.
- Caffeine hangs around in the body for several hours after consumption and even if it doesn't keep you up it can still interfere with the quality of your sleep. If you struggle with your sleep avoid drinking coffee and energy/caffeinated drinks after midday.
- Similarly, nicotine stimulates the central nervous system. If you do smoke, try to avoid doing so in the two hours before bed.
- Avoid alcohol in the two to three hours before bed. Alcohol is a sedative (it can make you fall asleep more quickly) but it blocks deep sleep. If you drink regularly, try to keep within the recommended alcohol limits and have at least two alcohol-free days per week (see page 122 for more on this).
- Don't take distractions into the bedroom. Remember, the bedroom is for sleeping and sex. If you struggle to sleep avoid taking any distractions (books, e-readers, smartphones, laptops) into the bedroom.
- Stop using light-emitting devices (smartphones, laptops, e-readers, etc.) at least an hour before bed. If you must be on a device be sure to switch it to night mode or download an app that filters out blue light.
- If you use your smartphone as your morning alarm, consider buying a separate alarm clock for this purpose. Failing that, turn your phone to silent and turn off social media notifications so that you are not disturbed by them.

Thinking

The fact that talking therapy is the recommended first-line treatment for insomnia both in the UK and US tells us that the major cause of insomnia is psychological. Sometimes the things that keep us up at night are normal features of life like adjustment to significant change or recovering from a break-up. Given a little time this tends to right itself (you may find Chapter 12 useful for advice on how to effectively manage these events) and you will return to your normal sleeping habits. But sometimes general worries can get in the way of a good night's sleep. If this sounds like you, consider the following tips:

- Everyday anxieties (a task you have to do the next day, items you need to remember) can be effectively managed with a worry book – keep a notebook beside your bed and write down any last-minute tasks or reminders that have a habit of cropping up just as you decide to go to bed. This way you can be reassured that you won't forget them but they won't be turning over in your mind all night.
- If you experience more prolonged worries, anxieties, negative thoughts or mood problems, a counsellor, psychologist or CBT-I trained practitioner may be able to help you.

Takeaways

- Adequate, good-quality sleep is *essential* for brain care and mental health. Addressing sleep issues and trying to restore natural sleep should be a priority for patients and mental health professionals.
- Watch out for sleep inertia! Leave at least 20 minutes between waking and doing a task that requires high levels of focus or accuracy.

- Aim to get at least 30 minutes of natural light in the morning or at lunchtime – this will help to anchor your circadian rhythm and promote healthy sleep.
- It may be worth trying to identify your BRAC. Use the tracker on page 313 to identify your ideal bedtime.
- If you are having trouble maintaining a healthy sleep pattern try working with a therapist trained in CBT-I or an evidence-based app like Sleepio.
- www.sleepstation.org.uk is an online CBT-I programme. Access is free for eligible NHS patients or available to purchase.

CHAPTER 7

Improving Your Brain Health through Nutrition

If I asked you which foods you should eat to look after your physical health you would probably be able to give me a pretty good list of candidates and healthy habits; eat plenty of fruit and veg, not too much sugar . . . that sort of thing. But most people don't know about the powerful role that nutrition plays in brain health and mental well-being. Yet, we experience the effects of foods on our brains every day. Whenever you have a cup of coffee or a couple of glasses of wine you soon feel the effects of nutrients on the brain. Caffeine makes you more alert, can improve attention and create positive feelings. Alcohol can make you feel more relaxed and, at higher concentrations, affects mental functions like perception, balance and mood. The thing about caffeine and alcohol is that their effects are acute; they can be felt immediately. Food is different. While food also has measurable effects on the brain, its impact is gradual, building up over time. This is why eating well for brain health isn't about quick fixes; it's about building up regular long-term habits.

People are often surprised to hear that although it only accounts for about 2–3 per cent of your total body weight, your brain makes up around 20–25 per cent of your daily energy requirement. It is punching well above its weight in terms of energy needs. But it's not just about the calories your brain needs to function optimally. From neurotransmitter production to action potentials, the brain uses vitamins and minerals in all of its cellular activity. All that activity creates a huge demand for nutrients and, if you start running low on those, your brain simply will not be able to function properly.

Since your brain is responsible for all your thoughts and feelings – all your best ideas – it makes sense that you should want to feed it properly. If you had a new puppy you would probably spend some time researching what the best food was for it. We rarely treat our brains with the same level of care. Until recently brain nutrition had not been taken seriously by mental health researchers (big mistake), but we now have strong evidence of the impact of food on our brains.

Food is one of the quickest and easiest ways to start improving your brain health and throughout this chapter I will give you the lowdown on foods to include in your diet to give your brain the best chance of staying fit. But first: a quiz!

Food frequency questionnaire
Grab a pen and fill in the following tables.

How often *on average* do you eat the following foods?

	Never	Less than once a month	1–3 times per month	Once a week	2–4 times per week	5–6 times per week	Every day
A bowl (80g) of dark green leafy veg, such as watercress, spinach, rocket, kale or chard (fresh or cooked)							
A palm-sized portion of oily fish, such as salmon, mackerel, anchovies, sardines, sprats, whitebait or herring (fresh, frozen or tinned)							
A mug-sized portion of berries, such as strawberries, blueberries, raspberries, blackberries or cranberries (fresh or frozen)							
A mug-sized portion of beans and legumes, such as baked beans, kidney beans, chickpeas (including hummus), butter beans or lentils							
A fist-sized portion of wholegrain foods, such as brown rice, wholewheat pasta, whole oats, barley or wholegrain sourdough bread							
A palm-sized portion of meat, such as chicken breast or leg, pork or lamb chop or beef steak							
Meat products, such as sausages, salami, chorizo, ham, bacon or burgers							
Sweet snack foods, such as chocolate bars, breakfast biscuits, granola/cereal bars, gummy sweets, a slice of cake or pie							

Vegetables from the onion family, such as onions, leeks, chives, shallots, spring/salad onions (scallions) or garlic							
Root vegetables, such as carrots, parsnips, swede, celeriac and Jerusalem artichokes							
Tea (green, white or black) or coffee							
Naturally or artificially sweetened beverages, such as cordial, iced coffee, ready-made drinks, energy drinks or sports drinks							
Raw unsalted nuts, such as Brazil nuts, almonds, hazelnuts and walnuts							

How often *on average* do you cook with the following foods?

	Never	Less than once a month	1–3 times per month	Once a week	2–4 times per week	5–6 times per week	Every day
Spices, such as cinnamon, coriander (seed), cumin, turmeric, chillies or paprika							
Herbs, such as parsley, rosemary, thyme or basil (fresh or dried)							
Cook or dress food with olive oil							

I've asked about these foods because they are the ones most strongly associated (positively or negatively) with brain health. For example, one recent study showed that older people who ate a daily serving of leafy green vegetables had slower rates of brain ageing: their brains looked and behaved as though they were 11 years younger!

We'll have a think about your answers in a moment. First, I want to tell you about some of the research.

Nutrition Research

Nutrition research is notoriously hard to do. People often don't remember what they have eaten accurately, and factors such as genetics and activity levels can vary the amounts of nutrients individuals need. To get a good sense of how diet affects mental health you have to start by observing large groups of people and looking at overall patterns.

A large (15,000 participants) Spanish study, which was the first to track people over 10 years, showed that diets high in nutrients are linked to a reduced risk of depression. The healthier your diet the less likely you were to develop depression over 10 years.

The researchers looked at three diets:

- Mediterranean diet: characterised by the consumption of vegetables, legumes, fruits and nuts, cereals, fish and seafood; a low intake of meat and dairy products; and moderate alcohol intake.
- Vegetarian dietary pattern: a kind of 'flexitarian' diet that promotes eating plant foods (including potatoes) most of the time, but allowing for a little meat.
- Healthy eating index: promotes eating larger amounts of vegetables, fruits, wholegrain bread, nuts, beans and pulses, omega-3s and unsaturated fats, and smaller amounts of

sugar-sweetened beverages and fruit juice, red/processed meat, trans fats and alcohol.

As part of the study, the researchers also looked at activity levels, body mass index (BMI), health history and vitamin supplementation, and the analysis was controlled for a number of variables including age, sex and smoking status.

The researchers looked at levels of adherence (how much each person stuck to any one of the three healthy diets) and the participants were split into five groups. On a scale of 1–5, those in Group 1 ate the least healthy diets while those in Group 5 were healthy eating gurus. The results showed that those in Groups 2–5 had a 25–30 per cent reduced risk of developing depression than those in Group 1. Interestingly, there was a plateau in this protective effect once the participants had moderately good diets. The researchers believed this to be due to a threshold effect; once you are eating enough of a nutrient there is no additional benefit of consuming larger amounts of it.

A British study that followed 10,000 civil servants over many years found that women with poorer diets were much more likely to develop recurrent depression.

These kinds of studies help us to understand relationships, but to be able to say that one thing *causes* another we have to test it. In 2017 a team of Australian researchers did just that.

The 'SMILES' Trial

The 67 participants in this 12-week study were depressed adults who had a clinically defined poor diet: one that was low in fibre, fruit and vegetables and lean protein, and high in sweets, salty snack foods and processed meats. Some participants were receiving treatment for their depression in the form of medication, talking therapy or both.

Participants were randomly assigned to either a nutritional intervention group or a befriending control group. In the intervention group the participants had seven one-hour sessions with a registered nutritionist who provided them with personalised nutritional advice and meal plans, and coached them around goal-setting and motivation to help them to stick to a Mediterranean-type diet.

In addition, participants were encouraged to reduce their intake of: ' "extras" foods, such as sweets, refined cereals, fried food, fast food, processed meats and sugary drinks (no more than three per week). Red or white wine consumption beyond two standard drinks per day and all other alcohol (e.g. spirits, beer) were included within the "extras" food group. Individuals were advised to select red wine preferably and only drink with meals.'

Those in the social support/befriending group had seven one-hour meetings with a trained professional who talked to them about neutral topics. Anxiety, depression and general mood were assessed at the beginning and end of the study, along with data such as weight, waist circumference, fasting blood glucose and cholesterol.

The results showed that people in the dietary intervention group were four times more likely to be in remission at the end of 12 weeks than those in the befriending group. They also had reduced severity of anxiety symptoms. There was no change in BMI, blood glucose, cholesterol or physical activity within or between the groups. This study has since been replicated by other teams with similar results. It tells us that, at least for some people, a poor diet contributes to their depressive symptoms.

We eat several times a day, which gives us many opportunities to choose foods that support our overall brain health. The food frequency questionnaire you completed on page 91 will give you a sense of where you are now. While there is no such thing as a 'perfect' diet, knowing which foods are good for the brain will help you to make more brain-healthy choices. So let's look at some foods in more detail.

Oily Fish and Seafood

What are they?
Anchovies, cockles, herring (including kippers and bloaters), mackerel, mussels, pilchards, salmon, sardines, sprats, trout, whitebait. Fish roe (not soft roe). Fresh, frozen, smoked, tinned.

What's the big deal?
Why is oily fish so important for your brain? Because oily fish *is* your brain. Kinda. When people talk about fats the terms 'saturated' and 'unsaturated' come up a lot. The level of saturation refers to the chemical structure of the fat. Generally speaking, saturated fats are solid at room temperature (butter, lard, dripping, coconut oil) and unsaturated fats, found in seed and nut oils and oily fish, are liquid at room temperature. Dairy foods contain a combination of saturated and unsaturated fats.

Oily fish contains particular types of unsaturated fats called 'essential fatty acids'. They are essential because your brain needs them for healthy function, but the body is unable to synthesise them. You must get these fats from the diet. But why are they so important?

Two kinds of essential fats in a family called 'omega-3' – eicosapentaenoic acid (EPA) and docosahexaenoic acid (DHA) – play particularly important roles in the brain because they form the cell membranes. They act like the exterior walls of a house, keeping what should be on the inside in, what should be on the outside out and only letting in desirable guests. If you are not getting enough of these fats in your diet it is as if, bit by bit, the bricks are being taken out of the walls. The house will be able to stay upright for a while but eventually it will start to break down. Alternatively, they may be substituted for other fats, which will negatively effect the function of the cell membrane.

DHA also helps to supports cell signalling, allowing brain cells to communicate with each other, while EPA reduces inflammation. A lack of DHA has a detrimental effect on the brain as can be seen in the pictures below:

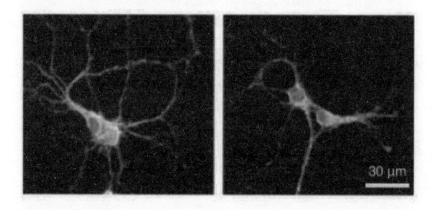

On the left is a mouse neuron that has had sufficient omega-3. It has a lot of strong, active connections. On the right, the brain cell deprived of omega-3 has 50 per cent fewer connections. Omega-3s have been shown to upregulate hippocampal neurogenesis and consequently have been linked to reduced depression risk. Older adults with diets rich in these fats have brains that age more slowly than those who do not.

There is a third brain-essential fat called α-Linolenic acid. We'll talk more about that on page 103.

How to eat them

- Reprise a classic – tinned sardines on toast is a classic snack or light meal. If you combine them with wholegrain toast you'll get the added fibre benefits.
- Tinned sardines also feature in one of my favourite pasta dishes. Warm the sardines in a tomato-based pasta sauce and then stir in your cooked wholewheat pasta. Sprinkle with garlic breadcrumbs for a delicious, satisfying, brain-healthy dish.
- Add salmon or trout to a fish pie.
- Make your own mackerel pâté by whipping smoked mackerel with a little cream cheese and black pepper.
- Try a fish stew. Fry chopped onion, carrots and celery in olive oil until soft. Add 2 tablespoons of tomato purée and 2 cloves of crushed garlic. Add about 200ml of fish stock or water, a bay leaf, pepper and some chilli flakes. Simmer for 10 minutes and then add pieces of white fish, salmon/trout and some mussels. Pop the lid on and simmer until the fish is cooked. Check the seasoning, sprinkle with chopped parsley and serve with crusty bread to soak up the sauce.
- Vegans can ensure that they get their regular intake of these essential fats by taking an algae-based omega-3 supplement.

What about meat?

Dietary recommendations about meat are often conflicting. National health guidelines in the UK recommend that people reduce their meat consumption to reduce risks associated with heart disease and bowel cancer. However, a controversial new international meta-analysis has reported that the evidence on which that information is based may be of low quality.

In clinical trials vegetarianism has been associated with an increased risk of mood disorders. This could be for number of reasons including the nutritional content of vegetarian diets, personality traits linked to vegetarianism, and the fact that most vegetarians are women and women have a higher risk of mood disorders.

People who eat a lot of red meat (beef and veal, pork, lamb and mutton, goat and venison) tend to have higher rates of certain cancers, but there may be other factors at play. It is also very hard to disentangle meat consumption from other nutrients in the diet. Do people who eat a lot of red meat tend to pair it with fries and a sugary drink, or a salad and a piece of fruit? Increasingly we are understanding that it is the *overall diet quality* that impacts health (including brain health) rather than individual foods.

What is clear though is that red meat production, especially beef, has environmental consequences, particularly in relation to the amount of land required to raise cattle. There are also important concerns about animal welfare in industrial farming.

At the moment it seems that there may be no specific mental health risks of eating meat as part of a well-balanced omnivorous diet. If you choose to eat meat it might be a good idea to focus on the *quality* of the meat that you consume. That may mean eating meat less often but choosing free-range and organic cuts purchased from a local butcher or delivered from a farm service, if that is available to you. If you do wish to cut back on red meat, you could try alternatives like poultry (chicken, turkey, goose, duck, game birds), eggs (a good source of brain-healthy B vitamins and choline) or vegetarian sources of protein such as tofu, seitan or beans.

Leafy Greens

What are they?

Beetroot tops, Brussels tops, chard, chicory (aka endive), collard greens, dandelion greens, kale (curly and cavolo nero), radicchio, rocket (aka arugula), Romaine lettuce, savoy cabbage, seaweed (nori), spinach, turnip greens, watercress.

What's the big deal?

As I mentioned earlier, leafy green vegetables are brain-protective. This is because of the wide range of brain-essential bioactive nutrients they contain such as:

Beta Carotene	Modulates the growth of new brain connections. Involved in brain cell survival and neuroplasticity. Promotes the production of neurotransmitters.
Folate	Reduces inflammation. Regulates gene expression (turning genes on or off). Improves cognitive function.
Vitamin K	Linked to better memory. Lower risk of dementia.
Lutein	May act as an antioxidant in the brain. Higher concentrations are linked with better cognitive function. Also protects eye health and prevents a degenerative eye disorder called 'age-related macular degeneration'.
Magnesium	Prevents synaptic loss. Required for over 300 enzyme reactions in the body (nearly every action in your body depends on enzyme action).
Potassium	Needed for nerve signalling. May help prevent the onset of Alzheimer's disease.

The research suggests that aiming for a serving of greens (one serving is equal to one cereal/dessert bowl of salad leaves or four tablespoons of cooked spinach/kale) every day is best for brain health. I know that sounds daunting, especially if you're not a fan of the green stuff, but I have a few suggestions that might help make it a little easier for you to incorporate these versatile vegetables into your regular routine.

How to eat them

- Frozen spinach is your friend. A bag of spinach in your freezer is a stealth nutrition hero. Frozen spinach comes in portion-sized chunks (two per person, please) and you can add them to *everything*: smoothies, soups, pasta sauces, pasta, rice (while it's cooking), curries, mash, hummus . . . And the magic of it is that it won't change the taste of the food much, so even if you hate the fresh stuff you can sneak it in and show your brain a little love.
- Buy a bag of mixed watercress, spinach and rocket and keep it in the fridge at home or work. Add a handful to your lunchtime salad or sandwich. A fresh bag will keep fine for the day if your job is mobile (taxi or bus drivers, for example). At home, put a handful in a bowl, dress with a little olive oil and salt and eat it as a 'starter' to your dinner.
- If you are a fan of Greek cuisine, then spanakopita should be top of the list. This delicious filo pie is filled with mixed greens and feta. Served with some cherry tomatoes and hummus this is a great brain-friendly meal.
- Romaine and cos lettuce are also delicious cooked. Cut into wedges and griddle in a hot pan for a couple of minutes until they get a little colour. Sprinkle with salt and olive oil before serving.
- Roast wedges of savoy or pointed cabbage in a hot oven for

about 20 minutes until brown around the edges and tender on the inside. Serve with a pesto dressing.

Nuts and Seeds

What are they?

Nuts: almonds, Brazil nuts, cashews, hazelnuts, peanuts*, pecans, pistachios, walnuts. Unroasted and unsalted.

Seeds: chia, flaxseed (aka linseed), hemp, poppy, pumpkin, sesame, sunflower. Unroasted and unsalted.

What's the big deal?

Seeds, nuts and nut butter have enjoyed a lot of popularity with fitness enthusiasts over the last few years due to their protein content.[†] But nuts and seeds are a key contributor to brain fitness too. They are rich in the other essential fat – α-Linolenic acid (ALA) – and polyphenols, powerful plant chemicals that, when digested by our gut microbes, produce phenolic acids that protect the brain by reducing inflammation and oxidation. They also help to improve how brain cells communicate and promote neurogenesis. Nuts and seeds are also a good source of antioxidant vitamin E, which has been consistently linked with better memory function in older age.

A nutrition study that lasted 20 years assessed how often women consumed nuts. When the 15,000 participants reached 70 years old, they completed repeated tests of their cognitive function. They

* Technically, peanuts are legumes, members of the bean family (see page 108).
† Nut and seed milks are a growing trend for people who wish to consume less dairy. However, they tend to be mostly water and do not contain the concentration of nutrients found in the whole food. You are free to enjoy them but they would not count as a 'serving' of nuts.

found that women who ate nuts five times a week had better brain function than those who did not eat them.

How to eat them
- Mixed nuts make a great snack. Two to three tablespoons is roughly one portion.
- If you already eat peanut butter, play around with different types of nut butters – almond, hazelnut and cashew are all available in most large supermarkets. You can also make them at home by blending raw or roasted nuts in a food processor until they form a paste.
- Use nut butters as the base for sauces and dressings, or try them in African peanut soup, a warming spicy soup that uses peanut butter as the base (try searching for a recipe online).
- Sprinkle chopped nuts or mixed seeds over porridge to get your day started on a brain-healthy note.
- A serving of mixed seeds sprinkled over a salad will add flavour and texture.
- Choose seeded wholemeal breads for an added fibre boost.

Berries

What are they?
Blackberries, blackcurrants, blueberries, cranberries, cloudberries, gooseberries, lingonberries, mulberries, raspberries, redcurrants, strawberries. Honorary mention for cherries and pomegranates, olives and olive oil.

What's the big deal?

Some of the most exciting research in Nutritional Psychiatry comes from the profound acute and long-term effects of berries on the brain.

The equivalent of 200g of fresh blueberries (they used freeze-dried ones in the study) increased blood levels of BDNF an hour later and immediately improved attention and short-term memory. In another study 200g of fresh blueberries resulted in improved word recall in children, and improved their accuracy on tests. Blackcurrants improved attention during a long, cognitively fatiguing task and cherries are linked with better mental flexibility, the ability to switch from one task to another. Another trial found that pomegranate anthocyanins (the compounds that makes them red) protected against memory deficits and improved memory retention six weeks after consumption. What else do you need to know to convince you to eat them?

How to eat them

You don't need any help from me on this one. Berries can be enjoyed fresh as a snack, a light dessert, with yoghurt/kefir and granola for breakfast and in smoothies. In Scandinavia they make berry soup topped with toasted oats for breakfast. Frozen berry mixes are a great cheaper option, and are just as nutritious.

Herbs and Spices

What are they?

Herbs: bay leaf, basil, chervil, coriander (leaves and stalks), curry leaves, dill, lavender, lovage, marjoram, mint, oregano, parsley, rosemary, sage, sorrel, tarragon, thyme.

Spices: allspice, black pepper, caraway, cardamom, cassia/cinnamon, cayenne, chilli, clove, coriander (seed), cumin, fenugreek, galangal, ginger, horseradish, lemongrass, mace, mustard, nutmeg, paprika, saffron, star anise, turmeric, vanilla and wasabi.

What's the big deal?

You will have noticed that coffee shops all over the country now offer a turmeric latte. This is a version of 'golden milk', a spiced milk drink that has been consumed in South East Asia for centuries. Turmeric's popularity comes from its status as an anti-inflammatory food. While most of the trials on turmeric supplements have been inconclusive, one consistent finding is that people who live in South East Asia have lower rates of dementia than those in the West, which researchers put down to their regular intake of a variety of spices that are a key feature of their cuisine.

Researchers are currently looking into the role of saffron, turmeric, pepper, ginger and cinnamon as potential anti-Alzheimer agents. Rosemary has long been associated with memory performance and a recent study has shown that consuming a rosemary extract can indeed improve memory. But it's not about taking isolated supplements; whole herbs and spices contain thousands of chemical compounds that may improve mood, slow brain ageing, improve blood flow, promote neurogenesis and inhibit neuroinflammation. So the key is to include small amounts of these foods into your everyday diet.

How to eat them

- Include herbs in your salad to add an additional dimension of flavour and nutrients.

- Add mixed fresh chopped herbs to your next omelette.
- Make a fresh pesto by blending a bunch of soft herbs (traditionally basil, but parsley works well too) with a clove of garlic, olive oil, a small handful of nuts (almonds, hazelnuts and walnuts are good) and season with salt and pepper. You can add some grated parmesan cheese too, if you like it.
- Use fresh mint or rosemary steeped in hot water to make a refreshing hot drink.
- Make a salsa verde. Translating as 'green sauce' this combination of chopped herbs, vinegar and oil is delicious on almost any savoury dish – fish, chicken, steak, tofu, roasted vegetables, rice and couscous. Make a batch and keep any extra in the fridge.
- Tabbouleh is a salad made with bulgar (a type of wheat), tomatoes and lots of fresh chopped herbs. Try serving it with chicken, fish or tofu.
- Explore Asian cuisine. Many spices are native to the tropical regions of South East Asia so this way of cooking naturally incorporates these wonderful ingredients. Set yourself a challenge to cook one new Asian dish a month to get into the habit of cooking with spices.
- If you make coffee in a cafetière, on the stove or using a filter, try adding a quarter of a teaspoon of mixed spices (ground cloves, cinnamon and nutmeg) to the ground beans for a warming spiced coffee. This is one of my favourite ways to get a regular dose of powerful plant polyphenols.

Beans, Alliums, Wholegrains and Cold Carbs

What are they?

Beans: adzuki, black, black-eyed, broad (aka fava), chickpea (aka garbanzo), kidney, lentils, lima, mung, peas, pigeon, pinto, runner, urad. And, technically, peanuts.

Alliums: chives, garlic, leeks, onions, shallots, spring onions (aka scallions or salad onions).

Wholegrains: barley (pot not pearl), buckwheat, bulgar, cornmeal or polenta (not cornflour), couscous (wholewheat), farro, freekeh, kamut, millet, oats (whole, including oatmeal and oat bran), popcorn, rice (brown, wild, red and black), rye flakes, spelt.

Cold carbs: cooked and cooled carbohydrates like cold pasta salad, sushi, pre-cooked* or fried rice, and potato salad. Honorary mention for mushroom.

What's the big deal?

I've put all of these ingredients together because, as far as your brain is concerned, they have one thing in common: prebiotics. We've long known that fibre is good for our bodies, helping to reduce the risk of bowel cancer for example, but what could this unloved nutrient do for your brain? It turns out, an enormous amount and it has everything to do with your gut.

The gut microbiome is the term for the wide variety of microbial species (bacteria, archaea, fungi, viruses, etc.) that live in our gut. Thankfully, they are not living there rent-free; they earn their

---

* Rice that stands for too long at room temperature can be a risk for food poisoning. If you are cooking a batch of rice for later use, cool it immediately in a shallow dish, and transfer to the fridge. Do not store for more than a day and do not reheat rice more than once.

keep by playing hugely important roles in our physical and mental health.

Firstly, they help us to digest our food, extracting energy and important nutrients. They even *make* some vitamins for us. They also synthesise a number of important compounds, such as short-chain fatty acids and neurotransmitters that influence brain function. See the following table for some examples:

Gut bacteria species	What compounds do they produce?	Effects on the brain
Streptococcus, Escherichia, Enterococci, Enterococcus, Lactococcus, Lactobacillus	Serotonin	Neurotransmitter important for emotion regulation
Lactobacillus, Bacillus	Acetylcholine	Important for learning and memory
Bacteroides, Bifidobacterium, Propionibacterium, Eubacterium, Lactobacillus, Clostridium, Roseburia, Prevotella	Short-chain fatty acids (SCFA)	Provide energy, regulate function of the gut lining, reduce inflammation
Escherichia, Bacillus, Lactococcus, Lactobacillus, Streptococcus	Dopamine	Important for regulating movement. Dysfunction linked to Parkinson's disease, Alzheimer's disease and depression

(Source: Alkasir, R., Li, J., Li, X., Jin, M. and Zhu, B., 2017. Human gut microbiota: the links with dementia development. *Protein & Cell, 8*(2), pp.90–102)

But perhaps the most important job for the gut microbiome is its responsibility for modulating immune function. Around 70 per cent of the lymphocytes (a type of white blood cell) that circulate in the body are found in the gastrointestinal tract. A healthy gut microbiome teaches the immune system how to distinguish which substances are friends or foes. Studies have shown that introducing infants to peanuts early helps to train their immune systems to recognise peanut protein as harmless and reduces the likelihood that children will go on to develop nut allergies. There is even a recently discovered link between the immune system and childhood leukaemia. Researchers hope that eventually they could find the right combination of friendly bacteria that children could take in a milk drink to help reduce the chances of developing the disease.

Much of the unhelpful inflammation that we want to reduce starts in the gut. Part of that is a natural response: you become slightly inflamed every time you eat because food is one of the most common carriers of harmful bugs (e.g. spoiled meat) and your body wants to be ready. But the major cause of chronic inflammation in the gut is a lack of dietary prebiotic fibre.

Fibre (and the resistant starch found in cooled carbs and mushrooms*) is the favourite food source of the gut microbiome. If you are not getting enough fibre in your diet they effectively begin to starve. Faced with this situation your gut bugs turn to a backup fuel source called 'mucin'. Unfortunately, mucin forms the protective mucus layer that coats the inside of

---

* When starch is cooked and then cooled (e.g. for sushi) the chemical structure changes making it less digestible by the body but perfect food for gut microbes.

your gut. If your gut bugs eat through it, the tight cell junctions in the gut wall can open and become permeable. When this happens, bacteria and food molecules from the gut can enter the bloodstream (where they definitely don't belong). Seeing these intruders in the bloodstream, your immune system launches an attack and if this goes on for a long time you are likely to be in a state of chronic inflammation. As this blood flows through the brain it can trigger neuroinflammation, which we definitely want to avoid.

Gut Barrier Junction

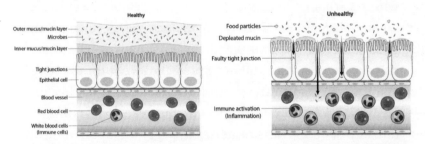

If you really want to take care of your brain, prebiotics (fibre and resistant starch) should be a high priority. And a wide variety of fibres are needed to cater to all the different microbial species.

How to eat them
- Make wholegrain your default – try to have wholemeal bread and pasta as your everyday choice, and keep the more refined white versions for when you have a real craving or a recipe specifically calls for them.
- Switch your normal baked beans for the mixed bean variety to increase diversity.

- Make a big batch of bean soup or bean chilli at the weekend and have it for lunch during the week.
- Make a pilaf. Combine cooked brown rice with chopped nuts, a tin of beans or lentils (drained), chopped fresh herbs and roasted vegetables. Dress with lemon juice and olive oil and serve with oily fish. Mixing any leftover pilaf with leafy greens makes a great lunch for the next day.
- You can buy pouches of precooked beans and grains. They cook in one minute and make a great fibre-rich lunch in moments.
- Roasted onions are a cheap and delicious side dish that works with almost anything savoury.
- Potato salad and pasta salad (homemade or shop-bought) are good sources of resistant starch. Even better if you leave the skins on the potatoes and use wholewheat pasta. Serve with oily fish and some leafy greens for a good all-round meal.
- Sushi and poke bowls also provide a good combination of resistant starch, oily fish and nutritious greens.

The gut–brain axis

The gut–brain axis describes the close connection and interaction between the brain and the gut. These streams of communication and influence are bidirectional i.e. the brain can influence the gut and what happens in the gut can literally shape the brain, both directly and indirectly.

Direct

- The vagus nerve (see Chapter 10) is thought to be the primary mode of direct action between the gut and the brain. In fact, there is growing evidence that neurological disorders such as Parkinson's disease and multiple sclerosis might start in the gut.

- Activation of the sympathetic nervous system (stress) can slow gut motility as blood is directed away from the gut to the limbs, or trigger gut symptoms, as seen in IBS.
- Difficulties of emotion regulation may manifest as problems with food, such as restrictive or binge eating.

Indirect

- The gut microbiome synthesises several compounds that travel to the brain in the bloodstream, cross the blood–brain barrier and influence brain health and activity.
- Immune and inflammatory activity in the gut can increase systemic inflammation, which may harm the brain.
- Problems with digestion or absorption may deplete the brain of important nutrients needed for proper function.
- Increased appetite is a common side effect of many antipsychotic medications.

Tea, Coffee and Cocoa

What are they?

Tea: various preparations of the *Camellia sinensis* plant: black tea, green tea, kombucha, matcha, white tea.

Coffee: prepared from roasted coffee beans, the seeds of berries from the *Coffea* species.

Cocoa: various preparations of the dried and fully fermented seed of *Theobroma cacao*, including cacao, cacao nibs, cocoa powder and dark chocolate.

What's the big deal?

Most of us are familiar with these three foods, typically consumed as beverages or confectionary. But these fermented foods have important brain-protective properties. This is due to them all being rich sources of polyphenols, which can enhance the elasticity of blood vessels, allowing blood to flow more freely. Polyphenols also feed the gut microbiome, which converts them into phenolic acids that are neuroprotective. Tea has been shown to reduce anxiety and improve memory and attention, and while some active compounds have been identified, the best effects are seen when tea is consumed as a whole food (i.e. not just the L-Theanine supplement). Coffee lovers will be pleased to hear that caffeine boosts the levels of an enzyme in the brain that has been shown to protect against dementia. And dark, polyphenol-rich chocolate has been shown to increase blood flow to the brain and improve working memory and visual function.

How to eat them

- Two to three cups of coffee and nearly unlimited tea per day has been shown to be neuroprotective, just watch any added sugar.
- Add a green tea bag to the pan when you boil water for pasta or rice. You won't taste it, but you'll be getting an extra hit of polyphenols. Discard the tea bag after cooking.
- To get the most benefits, chocolate should be dark: 70 per cent cocoa solids or above.

- Sprinkle cacao nibs on nut butter toast or vanilla ice cream for a little crunch and a nutritional boost.
- Try matcha, ground whole leaf green tea. Add a pinch to smoothies. (Although it is expensive so it's not an essential item.)

Water

It would be remiss not to also mention hydration. Your brain is around 80 per cent water and even small percentage drops in hydration are associated with increased fatigue, poorer cognitive function and worse mood. People often do not notice how thirsty they are, so a visual cue can be helpful. Place a refillable bottle on your desk, or wherever you spend most of your time. Having water in easy reach will help to keep you effortlessly hydrated.

Vitamin D

The emphasis throughout this chapter has been on the benefits of whole foods and overall dietary pattern rather than individual nutrients. That's because this is how we eat and how we have eaten for thousands of years. As such, this is how your body has evolved to digest and utilise nutrients. Moreover, though we have been able to isolate many of the nutritional components in foods, there are still hundreds of compounds, particularly in plants, that scientists have yet to identify. These undiscovered nutrients are likely to be responsible for many of the brain-health benefits associated with these foods. The message from nutritional science is loud and clear: get your nutrients from a varied, balanced and enjoyable diet composed primarily of unprocessed or lightly processed foods.

Furthermore, recent reviews and meta-analyses have concluded that, for people without a deficiency, there is little value in taking vitamin supplements. One exception to this rule is vitamin D. Vitamin D is a steroid hormone (the same family as cortisol, oestrogen, progesterone and testosterone), which modulates the activity of the immune system. If you are worried about having low levels of oestrogen or testosterone, you should take your vitamin D status as seriously. In 2016 the UK government's Scientific Advisory Committee on Nutrition (SACN) published a review of the evidence of the role of vitamin D on health, concluding that about a quarter of UK adults were deficient in vitamin D, with this number increasing to 40 per cent during winter, and rates of deficiency were higher in darker skinned people and those who spent more time indoors.

A small trial of older adults with deficient levels of vitamin D suggested that supplementation seemed to increase clearance of amyloid beta from the brain (remember that a build-up of amyloid is one of the key features of Alzheimer's). Sufficient vitamin D may also help to upregulate neurotrophic factors (neurogenesis) and support neuronal survival.

The UK's Department of Health now recommends that people with white skin consider taking a daily supplement containing 10 micrograms of vitamin D during the autumn and winter. Higher risk groups (people who are housebound, who cover most of the skin when outdoors, and those of Asian, African or Afro-Caribbean descent) should consider supplementing year-round.

Now you know why these foods are so important, what does a brain-healthy dietary pattern look like? The diet in the SMILES Trial (see page 95) looked like this:

- Whole grains (5–8 servings per day; 1 serving = 2 heaped tablespoons)
- Vegetables (6 servings per day)
- Fruit (3 servings per day, especially berries)
- Legumes/beans (3–4 servings per week)
- Low-fat and unsweetened dairy foods (2–3 servings per day)
- Raw and unsalted nuts (1 serving per day)
- Fish (at least 2 servings per week)
- Lean red meats (3–4 servings per week)
- Chicken (2–3 servings per week)
- Eggs (up to 6 per week)
- Olive oil (3 tablespoons per day)
- Wine (up to 2 standard glasses per day, ideally red)
- 'Extras': sweets, refined cereals, fried food, fast food, processed meats and sugary drinks (3 servings per week)

Now have a look at your answers from the 'food frequency questionnaire' on page 91. How close do you fall to these recommendations? Of course, this is not a strict protocol; you don't have to be 100 per cent spot on, after all, you are not a robot. Just use these guidelines to tailor your food intake to your personal tastes and lifestyle. You would be doing your Future Self a huge favour by trying to incorporate more brain-protective foods into your diet on a regular basis. Aiming to be one portion either side of the recommendations most of the time would be a great idea.

Vegan brain health

More and more people are moving away from eating animal foods for health, ethical or environmental reasons. While many people thrive on vegan diets, it is important to note that there are a few nutrients crucial for brain health that are very difficult to attain from plant foods alone. They are vitamin B12, the omega-3 fats EPA and DHA, and choline.

Vitamin B12 is found primarily in animal foods – fish, meat, poultry, eggs, milk and milk products. Non-animal sources include fortified foods and yeast extracts, such as Marmite. Spirulina, nori and barley grass are *not* reliable vegan sources of B12. Insufficient B12 damages the protective layer that insulates nerve axons (myelin) and B12 is also a necessary component of metabolism for every cell in your body, and for producing DNA.

The omega-3s DHA and EPA are major components of brain cell membranes and are anti-inflammatory. They are also important for heart health.

Choline forms the neurotransmitter acetylcholine, which has an important role in learning. It is found most abundantly in animal foods like liver, egg yolks and seafood. Choline can also be found in plant foods such as wheatgerm, peanuts and broccoli but in smaller amounts.

Deficiency

Deficiency symptoms of B12 can start out quite vague, with general fatigue and tiredness. Later symptoms include pins and needles, pain or numbness in the hands and feet, a sore tongue, mouth ulcers, muscle weakness, disturbed vision, depression, confusion, poor memory, and problems with understanding and judgement. At its worst, B12 deficiency mimics dementia. Low choline intake is associated with poorer brain function and slower processing speed in children, and we have spoken about the importance of essential fats for brain health on page 97.

Omega-3 deficiency may show up as rough, scaly skin or dermatitis. People deficient in omega-3 who are given a supplement perform better on cognitive tests, but you are unlikely to notice this impairment as it happens gradually.

Choline deficiency may lead to muscle or liver damage. However, it is rarely seen as most people consume some animal foods.

What to do

For adults, the NHS recommends an intake of about 1.5 microgram/day of B12. Vegans should eat fortified foods, such as cereals, some plant 'milks', meat substitutes and yeast extract, two or three times a day, or take a supplement to ensure adequate intake. An algae-based supplement can provide EPA and DHA for those on a vegan diet and, similarly, choline supplements are available in most health food stores.

Bite-Sized Changes

If you have eaten a not-so-great diet for a long time the idea of changing can seem really daunting, but it needn't be a total pain. First of all, I am not asking you to cut anything out completely. You can see in the SMILES Trial that participants were able to eat 'extra' foods every other day or so and still saw improvements. For the most part, the benefits in nutrition come from what you *add in* rather than what you take out. So think about the ways that you can add the protective foods – oily fish; vegetables including dark leafy greens; fruit, including berries, apples, pears and bananas; nuts; wholegrains; herbs; spices; tea and coffee – into your current meals:

- Smoothies are one of the easiest ways to combine a lot of brain-healthy ingredients:
  - Try your choice of milk with 1 banana, 30g wholegrain oats (or other wholegrain flake), 1 tablespoon nut butter and 1 tablespoon cocoa powder for a delicious breakfast smoothie.
  - Fresh or frozen spinach added to smoothies hardly affects the taste but provides a daily dose of greens.
  - Sprinkle smoothies with some mixed seeds for a bit of crunch.
- Subscribe to a veg box. They usually provide a wider variety of veg than you would normally buy and encourage you to eat more seasonally. Knowing that another box is arriving in a few days encourages you to find creative ways to increase your veg intake.

Dietary Inflammatory Index

The Dietary Inflammatory Index (DII) is a scale designed to classify whether a person's diet is broadly pro- or anti-inflammatory. The index has been used in numerous clinical trials, and the emerging consensus is that the higher inflammatory potential of a person's diet, the worse their brain function.

A large prospective study that included data from more than 26,000 people and followed them for an average of five years found that people with a more pro-inflammatory diet had a greater risk of developing depression. Further, higher scores on the DII are associated with:

- higher white blood cell count (a marker of inflammation) in people of average body weight
- higher blood levels of pro-inflammatory cytokines
- poorer academic performance in children
- greater risk of recurrent depression
- mild cognitive impairment and dementia in women, and poorer memory and overall cognitive performance in the elderly

According to the DII the foods and nutrients with the most anti-inflammatory potential are:

- beta carotene (found in brightly coloured vegetables)
- fibre
- flavones and flavenols (berries)
- garlic
- ginger
- green and black tea
- iron
- omega-3 fats (oily fish, seafood)
- turmeric
- vitamins A, C, D and E (fruit, vegetables, oily fish, nuts)

Foods to Limit

A handful of substances may present harm to the brain, particularly at higher doses, or in people who are sensitive to them. You may wish to limit your exposure to them, but please consult a registered nutritionist or dietitian before making any major changes to your diet to limit risk of nutrient deficiencies.

Alcohol

Alcohol is a prime example of the adage 'the dose makes the poison'. In small amounts – within or below the NHS recommendation of 14 units per week – and when not consumed in a binge-type pattern, it may be neuroprotective through hormetic, antioxidant and anti-inflammatory mechanisms. In fact, light-moderate drinkers seem to have less cognitive decline than non-drinkers. However, there is a tipping point at which alcohol becomes both acutely and chronically harmful for the brain. Alcoholic dementia, which may account for up to 10 per cent of all dementia cases, describes the shrinking of the brain caused by excessive alcohol consumption. Depending on the severity and chronicity of the damage, it may reverse when people stop drinking, but for many chronic alcoholics the damage is lasting.

The one caveat to the 'safe in moderation' message around alcohol is in pregnancy.

Foetal alcohol syndrome is a known risk when women drink during their pregnancies, which manifests in delayed development (lower birth weight, smaller head circumference), poor growth, learning difficulties and increased risk of psychological illness during adolescence and adulthood. The growing scientific consensus is that even occasional alcohol consumption during pregnancy may provoke harmful brain changes in children.

Caffeine

Caffeine, in people who can tolerate it, does not present a brain-health risk. In fact, it is associated with improved cognitive performance, reduced risk of dementia and even lower mortality. The cognitive risks of caffeine are associated with its detrimental effects on sleep quality. There is currently particular concern about children's consumption of caffeinated energy drinks and cola, particularly as sleep is so essential for learning and overall brain development. It is likely that many young (and not so young) people are stuck in a vicious cycle of staying up late working, watching TV or browsing online, getting insufficient sleep and compensating for daytime somnolence with caffeine in the day, which impairs sleep . . . Additionally, excess caffeine can exacerbate anxiety symptoms. Try to stick to having your last caffeinated drink before or around midday and maintain good sleep habits to mitigate these risks (see page 83).

Free and liquid sugars

Determining the impact of excess sugar in the diet is a difficult task because habitual overconsumption of sugar is typically accompanied by additional weight gain, which has its own brain-health risks independent of total sugar intake. Yet, animal studies indicate that high-sugar diets are linked to cognitive impairment, and insulin insensitivity/impaired glucose metabolism in the brain is a feature of Alzheimer's disease (see page 130).

Glucose is the preferential fuel source of the brain and is derived from the digestion of starchy food such as wholegrains and root vegetables. When glucose is consumed the brain recognises the intake of nutrients and satiety is increased i.e. you feel less hungry. Conversely, fructose (in the form of fructose-sweetened beverages, not whole fruit) bypasses this process, does not increase satiety and, therefore, is easier to overconsume. In addition, the influx of sugar in the form of sugar-sweetened beverages (SSBs) occurs much faster than the equivalent amount in the form of food. As such, the impact on blood sugar and metabolism is much more dramatic.

A double-blind randomised controlled trial found that just three weeks of low to moderate consumption of SSBs increased blood levels of the pro-inflammatory cytokine CRP by 60–109 per cent in healthy young men. In a separate cross-sectional (correlational) study, higher intake of SSBs was linked with lower brain volume and poorer cognitive performance. The researchers state that the effects on brain size of consuming one to two or more SSBs per day was equivalent to one to two years of brain ageing. In terms of actual performance on cognitive tests it was likened to having a brain that was 6–11 years older.

A government survey of the UK population reported that both adults and children are consuming too much free sugar. Free sugar is defined as:

- All monosaccharides (e.g. glucose and fructose) and disaccharides (e.g. sucrase and lactose) added to foods by the manufacturer, cook or consumer, plus sugars naturally present in honey, syrups and unsweetened fruit juices.
- Fruit purées and pastes, and vegetables in puréed and juice form.

It is recommended that free sugars not comprise more than 5 per cent of the daily energy intake for anyone over the age of two. However, most people consume at least twice this amount, with sugary cereals, confectionary and non-alcoholic beverages accounting for most of the sugar in people's diets. In fact, a single can of sugar-sweetened soda can include at least this amount of sugar, meaning that any additional free sugars eaten that day would take you over the recommended healthy limit.

Artificial sweeteners

Concerns over the potential health risks of high levels of sugar consumption have driven growth in the number of food and drink products sweetened with artificial sugar substitutes such as aspartame, acesulfame K and sucralose. Some human research has suggested that artificial sweeteners may affect how the brain senses nutrients and some of these additives may trigger migraines in individuals sensitive to them. However, it is important to note that the European Food Safety Authority has assessed all of these products to be safe for human consumption at the average rates of habitual intake. So there is no conclusive human evidence suggesting that there are any direct brain risks associated with consumption.

However, some *in vitro* and animal trials have indicated that regular consumption of artificial sweeteners may adversely affect the gut microbiome, which, theoretically, could have knock-on effects on the brain. More studies are required to better understand whether there are any risks to human health.

Emulsifiers

Emulsifiers in foods are used to prevent fats and liquids in that food from separating, to retain moisture and to help create a smooth, rich mouth-feel in low-fat foods. Emulsifiers have been added to pre-packaged foods for decades, are subject to strict EU regulations and are 'generally recognised as safe' for human consumption in the amounts that they appear in the typical diet. There is increasing concern, though, that we have overlooked the potential harmful effects of emulsifiers on the important residents of our guts: the microbiota.

Mouse trials have demonstrated that relatively low levels of poly-sorbate 80 (P80) and carboxymethylcellulose (CMC) (provided in drinking water over 12 weeks) are associated with the degradation of the protective mucus layer of the gut and altered overall microbial composition, including reductions in bacterial species that are asso-ciated with health and increased levels of inflammation-promoting strains. In this study, administration of emulsifiers promoted low-grade inflammation in mice, and promoted colitis (gut inflammation) in strains of mice engineered to be vulnerable to the disease. It also elevated levels of lipopolysaccharide, the mole-cules that are found on the outside of bacteria, the same ones used to stimulate inflammation in human depression trials (see page 47).

Ex vivo trials (in which a substance is tested outside of the body) have demonstrated that P80 and CMC, when applied to a proxy of the human microbiome, altered its function in a pro-inflammatory direction.

Trials in humans are now underway to try to assess exactly what impact synthetic dietary emulsifiers might have on our microbi-omes and on our health. It is responsible that we wait until then to draw any conclusions. The prudent among you may want to limit the number of emulsifier-containing foods that you regularly consume, if that's possible for you.

A list of common emulsifiers is provided on page 315.

Antioxidant supplements

Many people will have heard about antioxidants, a class of compounds (including some vitamins) that neutralise reactive oxygen species (ROS). ROS are a natural by-product of metabolism but in excess they produce oxidative stress, which can damage DNA. The oxidative stress theory of ageing suggests that we age because of an accumulation of this oxidative damage, which has generated a lot of interest in antioxidant-rich foods and supplements. Some people have taken to daily regimens of high doses of these supplements in the hope of holding back the hands of time.

However, you will find few biologists who would endorse high-dose antioxidant supplementation. ROS are also produced by microglia as a defence against pathogens. They also act as signalling molecules that, kept in the right balance, are important for normal cellular function. So we are back to our conversation about balance.

An important example of this principle is the now (in)famous Beta-Carotene and Retinol Efficacy Trial (CARET) Study, an antioxidant treatment intervention for lung cancer. Since smoking creates elevated oxidative stress, which contributes to the development of cancer, and because people who eat plant-rich diets have reduced cancer risk, it was hypothesised that high doses of antioxidant vitamin A would protect individuals at high risk of developing lung cancer. However, in this randomised, double-blinded, placebo-controlled trial of over 18,000 people, those who received the supplements had a 39 per cent *increased* risk of developing cancer than people who received the placebo. And the cancers were more aggressive. The trial had to be halted because it was doing more harm than good. Sadly, people who had received the supplements remained at greater risk of developing cancer six years after the end of the study. One hypothesis is that the ingestion of high doses of exogenous antioxidants interfered with the body's own immune activity. ROS induce the death of precancerous cells, and the high dose supplements may have inhibited this action, allowing these cells to grow unchecked. More recently, a trial including more than 1,000 cancer patients found that antioxidant supplementation was associated with increased risk of cancer recurrence.

Nutritional scientists are still deciphering the myriad interactions between nutrients, immune cells, the microbiome and many other factors that influence nutrient-cell interactions. Until things are clearer, it may be wise to focus on acquiring your antioxidants from food such as berries, beans and dark leafy greens.

Coeliac or Gluten Psychosis

Coeliac disease (CD) is an autoimmune condition present in about 1 per cent of the population, in which the small intestine becomes inflamed in response to gluten. Over time, if the person continues to eat gluten-containing foods (wheat, barley, rye) the gut lining can be damaged, preventing nutrients from being absorbed, leading to malnutrition. Non-coeliac gluten sensitivity (NCGS) describes a syndrome in which people experience symptoms similar to CD but do not test positive for the disease. CD and NCGS are managed by maintaining a strict gluten-free diet.

Observational studies have recorded a higher risk of psychiatric and neurological disorders in patients with CD and NCGS, including problems with balance, epilepsy, depression, anxiety and schizophrenia. As far back at the 1960s there have been case studies in which psychotic symptoms have been reduced or resolved by eliminating gluten from the patient's diet.

Of course, it would be inaccurate to conclude that gluten is inherently psychoactive. If that were the case, nations with a high average intake of gluten (such as Italy) would have astronomically high levels of psychotic illness. In the same way that we don't demonise peanuts because some people are allergic to them, we need to take a rational view of gluten. It is currently understood that two factors have to coincide for the emergence of what is termed gluten psychosis:

1. Genetic vulnerability.
2. Compromised immunity, perhaps from an unrelated infection or illness, allowing gluten fragments to cross into the bloodstream or the brain, where they are recognised as 'foes' and trigger an inflammatory response. It is this immune activation that then precipitates the mental health symptoms.

It may be that for the rare individual who presents with rapid onset psychotic symptoms *and* gastrointestinal problems, trialling a medically supported elimination diet may prove helpful, if only to eliminate gluten as a potential culprit. However, as yet there is insufficient data to recommend that all patients with psychosis adopt a gluten-free diet. In relation to mental health, any dietary changes should be managed carefully, ideally with the support of a dietitian to ensure it does not create nutritional deficiencies.

Is Alzheimer's disease type 3 diabetes?

Your body has finely tuned mechanisms to keep its systems and internal conditions (such as blood pH, hydration and core temperature) in a fine balance. Diabetes mellitus is a metabolic disorder in which an individual's blood sugar is chronically and dangerously elevated, either through insufficient secretion of insulin or blunted insulin activity (insulin insensitivity). Insulin induces cells to take up glucose, either for immediate use or for storage.

Currently diabetes is delineated into two main types: 1 and 2 (T1DM and T2DM, respectively). T1DM is an autoimmune disorder that develops when the insulin-producing cells of the pancreas are destroyed, resulting in insufficient insulin production. T2DM is associated with diet and lifestyle, with a diet high in free sugars and low in fibre, and low levels of physical activity conferring increased risk of developing the disease. However, over the last two decades some researchers have suggested that Alzheimer's disease (or perhaps a subset of the disease) is in fact a type of diabetes of the brain.

Evidence in favour of this position comes primarily from epidemiological data that shows a relationship between T2DM and dementia risk, particularly vascular dementia. Further, individuals with T2DM are twice as likely to develop mild cognitive impairment, a common precursor to Alzheimer's, as those without diabetes.

One compound in particular, insulin-degrading enzyme, has been shown to be relevant to the disease progression of both diabetes and the accumulation of amyloid beta. However, a causative relationship has yet to be demonstrated.

While glucose metabolism is impaired in Alzheimer's disease, it is also true that obesity, a known risk factor for T2DM, is a condition of chronic low-grade inflammation and inflammation may independently lead to insulin insensitivity and cognitive impairment. Furthermore, insulin insensitivity can make blood vessels less flexible, which can reduce blood flow. Reduced blood flow may mean impaired delivery of nutrients and oxygen to the brain. Additionally, T2DM raises heart disease risk, and this damage to blood vessels may contribute to the incidence of vascular dementia.

Finally, other factors, such as sleep disorders and bacterial infection have been shown to influence Alzheimer's risk independently of insulin activity. The picture is complicated and there is certainly overlap between these conditions. However, as yet there is insufficient convincing evidence to form a scientific consensus. As such type 3 diabetes as a descriptive term for Alzheimer's disease remains controversial.

The evidence is clear and consistent that a healthy overall diet – one high in fruits (especially berries) and vegetables, wholegrains, oily fish, nuts, beans and olive oil, and lower in free sugars, processed meat and saturated fat – can protect against depression and dementia, and is associated with better brain functioning including better memory and improved attention, fewer brain lesions and increased neurogenesis.

Takeaways
- The brain is a highly metabolically active organ that needs a lot of energy, nutrients and hydration to function optimally.
- Immune function has direct and indirect effects on the brain. Nutrition and the microbiome influence the immune system.

- Overall eating patterns with lower pro-inflammatory potential
  are associated with better brain health in both the short- and
  long-term. Diets that are rich in fibre, diverse plant foods, nuts,
  beans and legumes, herbs and spices, olive oil and fatty fish are
  associated with lower systemic inflammation, and reduced risk
  and severity of depression and dementia.
- The brain can derive all the glucose it needs from the digestion
  of wholegrains and vegetables. Free sugars and sugar-
  sweetened beverages, fried foods and heavily processed foods
  should be eaten infrequently, ideally no more than three to five
  portions per week, if possible.
- Food is more than just the nutrients on our plate; it plays a
  central role in our social, cultural, religious and family lives.
  While I want you to eat well for your long-term brain health,
  you should also retain the freedom to enjoy food in these other
  important ways. Balance is the key. An obsession with 'healthy
  eating' (orthorexia) is just as detrimental to mental well-being
  as being malnourished.

CHAPTER 8

To Fast or Not to Fast

We have spent some time understanding the importance of proper nutrition on the structure and function of the brain. However, in recent years there has been a proliferation of public interest and scientific research into the potential health effects of food or energy restriction on human health. For decades researchers have noted that reducing energy intake (calories) by around 30 per cent of total daily requirement (while retaining protein, vitamin and mineral intake) can extend lifespan by up to 30 per cent depending on the organism.

Based on animal research, individuals across the world have started conducting their own experiments on the health benefits of caloric restriction (CR). While much of the emerging data is compelling in terms of the reduced heart disease risk, lower fasting glucose/insulin and increased insulin sensitivity, because we need to wait decades for the results we do not yet know whether humans will experience anything near the same level of life extension as seen in non-human animals. Additionally, long-term CR means that practitioners of this way of life are perpetually hungry, and few people are willing to make the trade-off for more years of life if those years are spent feeling a bit miserable because you never quite have enough food. There is also the risk of metabolic adaptation in the form of a slowed metabolic rate to compensate for the reduced energy intake. This might mean that, should these people return to a normal eating pattern, they would be more inclined to put on weight quickly and find it harder to lose.

In the last decade various fasting protocols have emerged as an alternative strategy to enjoy the benefits of CR without the constant hunger or the shifts in energy metabolism.

What Is Fasting?

Fasting is the act of going without food for a period of time. During these fasting periods individuals will typically consume only water or calorie-free beverages such as black tea and coffee or diet sodas. One of the difficulties in evaluating the research on fasting is that the terms are used interchangeably for a variety of different patterns (see below), so it can be difficult to establish a 'best practice'.

Type	Protocol	Detail
Time-restricted eating (TRE)	20:4 18:6 14:10	Practitioners aim to eat all of their daily meals/calories within a 'feeding window' of typically fewer than 10 hours. For example, 14:10 means fasting for 14 hours (this usually includes the overnight fast during sleep) and eating all meals within 10 hours. This may be achieved by delaying or skipping breakfast or having an early dinner.
Intermittent fasting (IF)	5:2	Individuals eat to their normal pattern for five days of the week and fast or significantly restrict food intake for two non-consecutive days.

Alternate day fasting Every other day fasting (EDOF)		Individuals alternate daily between their normal eating pattern and fasting or significantly restricting food intake.
Prolonged fasting		Food intake is completely restricted (only water is consumed) for a period of two or more consecutive days, typically three to five.
Fasting mimicking diet (FMD)	Prolon®	A patented, commercially available five-day meal plan of foods formulated to not trigger nutrient sensing pathways, allowing users to receive the reported benefits of prolonged fasting while being able to consume small amounts of food.

It may be that there is no best practice in relation to the range of fasting interventions, in the same way that there is no one diet that is suitable for every person on the planet. The research can provide us with broad evidence-based guidelines, but they must be tailored to the individual needs of each person.

Research evidence suggests that limiting the daily duration during which food is consumed can support physical health, independently of weight loss, but what about the brain?

Fasting and the Brain

Several clinical trials have demonstrated that a range of fasting protocols may have a beneficial effect on the brain through numerous mechanisms:

- A small preliminary trial on healthy lean men reported that levels of brain-derived neurotrophic factor (BDNF) in muscle tripled following a 48-hour fast. The increased availability of BDNF may confer brain benefits in terms of both neuroplasticity and cell survival.

- Fasting upregulates the production of ghrelin. Ghrelin is known as the 'hunger hormone' but it does more than just make you feel hungry. Animal trials have shown that ghrelin crosses the blood–brain barrier and increases neurogenesis in the hippocampus. Researchers speculate that this neurological action of ghrelin may account for the improved memory function associated with CR in humans.[*] Ghrelin may improve glucose sensitivity in some people. Ghrelin also upregulates the production and activity of orexin, a protein that activates dopaminergic, serotonergic and cholinergic brain cells, and thus plays a mediating role in mood and goal-driven behaviours. This action of ghrelin/orexin on mood may contribute to some reports of elevated mood during short periods of CR. However, over prolonged periods this apparent antidepressant effect may fade.

- Water fasting promotes rapid utilisation of stored glycogen and the transition to ketosis, a metabolic state in which fat rather than glucose is the main fuel source. The availability of this secondary fuel may be of particular relevance to individuals with impaired insulin sensitivity or elevated blood glucose.

- A handful of genes code for the production of a group of proteins called sirtuins, named SIRT1 to SIRT7. Numerous animal trials have demonstrated a life-extending effect of sirtuins, such that animals with gene variations that make

---

[*] CR also promotes insulin sensitivity and lowers levels of systemic inflammation, which may also contribute to the cognitive enhancements.

them produce a lot of sirtuin tend to live longer (though a few studies have disputed this). In humans, low levels of SIRT1 and SIRT3 correlate to disease progression in Alzheimer's disease. Furthermore, SIRT1 may be important for breaking down amyloid beta, the protein characteristic of Alzheimer's progression. Fasting stimulates the upregulation of SIRT1 and SIRT3, which may promote improved insulin sensitivity, the creation of new mitochondria and protection from stress and oxidative damage, all of which may contribute to better brain health.

- SIRT3 also upregulates a gene called FOXO3, which stimulates DNA repair. This is important because a build-up of DNA damage in nerve cells is linked with increased risk and severity of dementia including Alzheimer's disease.

As you can see, much of the evidence linking fasting and brain health is theoretical or still at the animal model stage. It is a little too soon to know how it might impact human brain health.

However, some fascinating discoveries in the world of fasting and human brain health have come from the laboratory of Professor Valter Longo at the University of California. In a 2014 paper Longo's team reported that a prolonged fast of more than three days stimulated the regeneration of damaged and aged immune cells upon refeeding, effectively 'refreshing' the immune system in humans. During the period of fasting the participants' white blood cell count dropped, indicating that the body was breaking down these cells to provide energy. Importantly, the cells that were prioritised for recycling were the damaged or older (senescent) cells. The body was effectively taking out the biological trash. Upon refeeding there was a spike in the number of a type of stem cell that makes a range of blood cells, including white blood cells and the old, damaged cells were replaced with fresh new ones.

Animal models suggest that a similar process of rejuvenation may also occur in nerve cells. The brains of mice placed on the equivalent of a three-day fast in humans were observed to shrink during the period of fasting, indicating that the same process of breakdown and recycling was occurring. Volume was restored after refeeding. Longo's lab is currently working on preliminary trials to assess whether fasting protocols have the potential to improve outcomes in neurodegenerative diseases such as multiple sclerosis in humans.

A word of caution

I would like to emphasise that the upregulation in stem cell production was seen on *refeeding* i.e. it is the intermittent nature of the fast that confers the benefit. Prolonged periods of extended fasting without careful refeeding will simply increase allostatic load – the 'wear and tear' on the body and the brain in response to stress. Animal models have shown that long-term CR or many days of fasting lead to negative shifts in neurochemistry and depressive symptoms that persist even after refeeding and weight normalisation. Additionally, long fasts promote chronically elevated stress hormones that have negative effects on brain health. In summary, it seems that occasional, short periods (12–24 hours) of reduced caloric intake may confer some brain-health and/or mood benefits, but can cause lasting damage if done for long periods (72+ hours) of time.

Who Should Not Fast?

One of the questions that has yet to be clearly established in the world of fasting is its suitability for women. Why should there be a difference in the effect of CR on male and female bodies? The short answer is: fertility and pregnancy.

Irrespective of an individual woman's conscious desire for children, her body is acutely sensitive to information from the environment about whether the conditions are suitable for pregnancy and child-rearing. For example, one of the key features of anorexia nervosa in women is amenorrhea, the loss or lack of a period. When a woman is taking in insufficient energy her body infers that it must be because there is not enough food available (i.e. famine conditions). During famine conditions infant mortality rates increase as do the risks of miscarriage and stillbirth. The evolutionary solution to mitigate these risks is to shut down fertility. However, hormones are multitaskers and the key fertility hormones also play a range of other roles in health and homeostasis (the process of keeping the whole body in a healthy balance). Thus amenorrhea and relative energy deficiency are associated with additional health risks linked to hormone imbalances, including lowered libido, acne, poorer mood and cognition, and osteopenia, the thinning of bones.

The available research indicates that overall energy balance is a crucial factor in regulating women's overall health, and this may function independently of body fat percentage. So an overweight woman who drastically reduces her energy intake may be at risk of hormonal dysregulation and negative health consequences, distinct from those associated with being overweight and obesity. And don't forget that psychological stress and excessive exercise can contribute to hormonal dysregulation, as any woman who has missed a period due to stress can attest.

So, the fasting landscape for women is a little more complicated than it is for men, and we are still waiting for more research to clarify the situation. Women wishing to attempt intermittent fasting would be prudent to focus on TRE, eating meals within a 10–12-hour window. They should pay particular attention to any effects on their menstrual cycle. If periods change in duration or regularity it would be wise to return to normal eating. It might also be prudent to assess hormones levels periodically to keep an eye on any sub-threshold hormonal changes that might affect fertility in the absence of changes in menstruation.

Aside from the potential safety risks for some women, as a clinician who works with people recovering from restrictive eating disorders, I hesitated about including this chapter. I am acutely aware of how well-intentioned relaying of fasting research can be misconstrued or misused in the service of these chronic and deadly illnesses. As such there are some important contraindications to trying this intervention.

You should not fast if:

- You know or suspect that you have a disordered relationship with food. This includes:
  - compensating for food intake with excessive exercise
  - feelings of guilt or self-loathing when you eat 'bad' foods
  - anxiety about food choices
  - regularly eating past the point of comfortable fullness (bingeing)

- purging behaviours such as vomiting or use of laxatives
- disconnection from your body's hunger and satiety signals i.e. not knowing if you are hungry or when you are full, not trusting those sensations
- You are in recent recovery from an eating disorder or disordered eating.
- You have a nutritionally poor diet. Fasting on a nutritionally poor diet will only deplete your body even more. You should focus on increasing the volume and variety of nutritional foods in your diet as a priority.
- You are chronically stressed and/or regularly sleeping fewer than seven hours per night. Again, fasting in these conditions will simply add to your allostatic load and is likely to do more harm than good.
- You are underweight, or fasting causes you to become underweight.
- You are pregnant.
- You exercise intensively or overtrain.
- You suffer from low blood pressure.
- Fasting makes you feel fatigued, shaky, nauseous or faint.
- Fasting impairs your sleep.
- You just don't like it.

As you can see, there are a lot of limitations. Essentially, you should be in a fairly good state of physical and emotional health before you consider adding any additional stress in the form of CR.

Fasting is not for everyone, and while every new dietary practice will have its proponents and even its zealots, it is important to remember that what works for someone else might not work – or even be good – for you. We all have different genetics, microbiomes, histories, energy demands and relationships with food, and these individual differences must be considered when we are thinking about changing the way that we eat.

If you try fasting and it makes you feel out of sorts, then stop. This is likely to be an important signal that, for your body, it is an excessive stress rather than a beneficial one.

Takeaways
- Human fasting research holds promise in relation to potential brain benefits, but it is still in its infancy and there is much that we still need to know about the long-term effects, both positive and negative, especially for women.
- Eating all of your daily meals within a 10–12-hour window seems to be a safe intervention for women wanting to access the potential benefits of elevated ghrelin and SIRT signalling.
- Listen to your body: if any fasting protocol makes your feel unwell or impairs performance, stop.

CHAPTER 9

How Physical Activity
Protects the Brain

Hopefully, it is becoming clear how dependent the brain is on the body for optimal function. It should come of little surprise that some of the most comprehensive and robust research that we have about which lifestyle factors have the most positive effect on the brain is from exercise and physical activity trials.

The research literature makes a distinction between physical activity (PA) – 'any bodily movement produced by skeletal muscles that requires energy expenditure' – and exercise – 'a sub classification of PA that is planned, structured, repetitive, and has as a final or an intermediate objective the improvement or maintenance of one or more components of physical fitness'.

So PA includes all movement, including walking to the shops and doing chores, whereas exercise is structured activity, such as going to the gym or for a run. I will refer to PA to cover both of these definitions, making the distinction between certain types of exercise where it is of particular relevance. A good rule of thumb is that any movement is beneficial and will give your brain a boost.

Aerobic or resistance

Aerobic activity includes activities that speed up your heart and breathing rate, while resistance activity is movements that help to strengthen muscle and maintain bone health.

Aerobic

- aerobics, water aerobics and step class
- cycling
- dancing and Zumba
- elliptical machine
- hiking
- ice or roller skating
- jogging/running
- Nordic walking and 'power walking'
- rowing
- skipping
- step machine
- swimming
- tennis

Resistance

- body weight exercises, such as push-ups, pull-ups, planks, squats, duck walks and exercises incorporating rubber resistance bands
- calisthenics
- free weight exercises incorporating dumbbells, barbells, kettlebells, medicine balls and weighted bags
- weight machines such as the leg press or squat rack

Combination

- boxing training
- circuit training
- climbing and bouldering
- CrossFit
- HIIT and circuit training class
- Vinyasa and rocket yoga

PA has been shown decisively to:

- reduce the risk of developing depression and anxiety, even when there is greater generic risk
- lower depression severity
- increase brain volume (delay and reverse brain ageing)
- reduce the risk of dementia
- improve memory, attention and accuracy
- elevate mood
- increase stress resilience
- improve academic achievement in children

In addition, exercise that includes an element of learning, like learning new moves in a dance class, provides an extra beneficial challenge for the brain.

How does PA confer all of these benefits? There are a number of ways, but the unifying principle is that the brain is an organ, which, like the other organs in the body, benefits from exercise. Whether it's bicep curls or a country walk, *movement protects the brain.* Let's look at some of the processes.

Brain blood flow

Aerobic exercise gets your heart pumping, delivering more oxygen and nutrients to hard-working muscles. But it is not just the muscles that benefit from this increased blood flow; brain blood flow (perfusion) increases during exercise too, which is associated with better cognitive performance, focus and attention immediately following the activity. Moreover, regular exercisers have higher resting brain perfusion than non- or intermittent exercisers. Annoyingly though, even elite athletes who take a break from training see a drop in resting perfusion (though they will have accumulated more benefits). It seems there is no shortcut: to keep your brain nourished you have to keep moving.

Neurogenesis

Brain-derived neurotrophic factor Brain-derived neurotrophic factor (BDNF) is the growth factor that promotes the growth of new brain cells and supports the survival of existing ones, especially in the hippocampus, the area of the brain important for memory. Low brain levels of BDNF are associated with depression and seen in neurogenerative disorders such as multiple sclerosis and Parkinson's disease.

Exercise robustly increases expression of BDNF. Thirty minutes of aerobic exercise can increase blood levels of BDNF by 30 per cent. These rises are linked to improvements on various tests of cognitive function, including memory and processing speed.

Expression of BDNF seems to follow a dose-response – the higher the intensity, the more BDNF rises. However, remember that at some point hormesis just becomes chronic stress (see page 65). Adequate rest and recovery is just as important as activity.

IGF-1 BDNF is not the only growth factor in town. IGF-1, the growth factor that stimulates hypertrophy (muscle growth) after exercise, is also involved in neurogenesis. Older women who participated in resistance training twice a week had fewer and smaller brain lesions (a marker of brain ageing associated with impaired cognitive performance) than women who resistance trained only once weekly.

Regular exercise is associated with greater hippocampal and overall brain volume. Since the brain naturally starts to shrink by 1–2 per cent per year starting around the age of 40, regular exercise can, in effect, reverse brain ageing. For the moment, exercise is the closest thing we have to the fountain of eternal youth.

Reduced inflammation

Although the physiological stress of PA leads to an acute increase in inflammatory markers, this is a hormetic response and, over the longer term, regular exercise is associated with low levels of systemic inflammation. Indeed, it is thought to be this reduction in inflammation that accounts for some of the recognised mood-enhancing effects of PA.

Furthermore, regular exercise stimulates the vagus nerve, which has a powerful anti-inflammatory effect. (See Chapter 10 for more on this.)

Absorbing neurotoxins

In Chapter 4, I described the kynurenine pathway (page 48). When the body is in a state of chronic inflammation, the amino acid tryptophan is co-opted away from the production of serotonin (the 'happy hormone') and melatonin (the sleep regulator) into the metabolic pathway for a compound called kynurenine, which is neurotoxic. So, you have two challenges: reduced availability of 'good' hormones and higher levels of brain-damaging kynurenine. Fortunately, when you exercise, kynurenine is absorbed from the bloodstream into the muscles so it has less opportunity to harm the brain.

Endorphins
PA, especially high-intensity exercise, can be really tough. Anyone who has done HIIT training or boxing fitness will know that pain of really pushing your physical limits. In response to this effort the brain releases endorphins, endocannabinoids and dopamine that produce feelings of pleasure and well-being. These chemicals are also linked to reduced anxiety and reduced sensitivity to pain.

Stress management
Cross-sectional research indicates an association between PA and lower levels of psychological distress. A survey of Scottish households found a dose-response effect: the more activity people engaged in the less stress they reported. In this trial it didn't matter what kind of exercise it was; all movement was associated with improvement.

Improved sleep
Regular exercise has been shown to improve sleep quality. We have already discussed in depth how crucial good sleep is for brain health (see Chapter 6) – exercise can help secure these benefits.

Body temperature

Exercise, particularly high-intensity PA, raises core body temperature, which can activate the production of heat shock proteins. Full details of the role these proteins play in brain health can be found on page 227.

How much exercise is enough?

- at least 150 minutes of moderate aerobic activity, such as cycling or brisk walking every week and
- strength exercises on two or more days a week that work all the major muscles (legs, hips, back, abdomen, chest, shoulders and arms)

Or:

- 75 minutes of vigorous aerobic activity such as running or a game of singles tennis every week and
- strength exercises on two or more days a week that work all the major muscles (legs, hips, back, abdomen, chest, shoulders and arms)

Or:

- a mix of moderate and vigorous aerobic activity every week – for example, 2 x 30-minute runs plus 30 minutes of brisk walking equates to 150 minutes of moderate aerobic activity – and
- strength exercises on two or more days a week that work all the major muscles (legs, hips, back, abdomen, chest, shoulders and arms)

(Source: NHS, 30 May 2018. Exercise. Retrieved from www.nhs.uk/live-well/exercise)

Why Yoga Works

Though all kinds of physical activity provide health benefits, the practice of yoga is a natural integration of many of the lifestyle factors that have been shown in clinical trials to promote brain health. In addition, a handful of clinical trials have shown yoga to be an effective and safe intervention for a range of conditions including depression, anxiety and IBS. Though I appreciate that yoga has a rich and ancient history rooted in spiritual development, I am referring here to yoga as most readers will know of it: the physical practice of postures (asanas), with a focus on breath, bodily awareness and meditation. Perhaps you have been unsure about trying yoga. Here is a brief overview of why yoga could be beneficial for mental health and why it might be worth a try.

Breath

One of the core features of yoga is the focus on controlled use of the breath. Transitions between postures are done in unison with the inhalation or the exhalation, such that, over time, the yogi comes to experience the body and breath moving as one. These breaths are typically deep, originating from the abdomen/diaphragm rather than the shallow breath of the upper chest, where many people habitually breathe. In addition, some yogis will utilise the ujjayi breath, an audible breath that is created by gently constricting the back of the throat. Many yoga instructors will also open and close their classes by leading the group in the chant of 'Om'. This mantra starts by taking a deep inhalation through the nose before enunciating the sound, which is completed with an extended 'mmm' that resonates through the mouth, throat and chest.

The resonant mantra, the deep diaphragmatic and ujjayi breath, with an emphasis on a long, slow exhalation, stimulates the vagus nerve, providing a powerful anti-inflammatory effect (see page 163). Furthermore, the focus on breathing through the nose that is typical of yoga can initiate a healthy pattern of brain activation, as we will see in Chapter 10.

Movement

The postures typically involve placing the body in positions that stretch or extend the muscles (e.g. 'downward dog'), holds and transitions that build strength (such as moving from plank to chaturanga) or balances. Stretching, at least in animal trials, has a demonstrated anti-inflammatory effect and, as noted earlier, body-weight resistance training upregulates the production of growth factors that promote the process of neurogenesis. Being able to retain good balance is associated with healthier ageing and may reduce the risk of falls as we age, which are a significant health risk for elderly individuals.

Meditation

The nature of the yoga practice – concentration on the breath, transitions to postures with a focus on alignment and the sensations within the body – takes attention away from nagging thoughts and incidental worries. Many teachers will actively orient their classes on mindfulness practices, such as separation from and observation of thoughts, or trying to focus on the space in between a thought (which is just as tricky as it sounds). Mindfulness and meditative practices are associated with reduced perceived stress, lowered anxiety, reduced inflammatory biomarkers and increased neurogenesis.

Compassion

The practice of yoga, and its broader spiritual tenets, focuses on developing compassion for yourself and others. Initially, this is through being mindful of how your body feels in the posture and not pushing against resistance or attempting to compete with someone else in the class. You may also be invited to 'dedicate' your practice; to keep someone in mind during the class whom you think may need some kindness. This principle extends to thinking about your interactions with other people, your impact on the world and the nature of your consumption.

There is a body of research demonstrating that compassion both for the self and for others is associated with greater resilience. More on this in Chapter 12.

Yoga as a powerful treatment intervention

The powerful anti-inflammatory and stress management effects of yoga have been demonstrated in clinical trials. One of my favourites is a recent study that compared the efficacy of yoga against a low FODMAPS diet for IBS. FODMAPS stands for 'Fermentable Oligosaccharides, Disaccharides, Monosaccharides and Polyols', which are types of prebiotics that can be fermented by the gut bacteria. FODMAPS are found in a range of plant foods, such as onions, garlic, beans, lentils, broccoli, apples and pears. You will notice that all of these foods feature highly on our lists of health-promoting and anti-inflammatory foods (see Chapter 7). However, in some people with IBS, the fermentation of FODMAPS and the gas produced can exacerbate gut symptoms. One effective treatment for IBS is to remove or radically reduce foods containing high amounts of

---

FODMAPS for a short while to give the gut a break before reintroducing them (because they are beneficial for the gut microbiome).

This study randomly assigned IBS patients to receive either a low FODMAPS diet or to attend two yoga classes per week for 12 weeks. At the end of the three months both groups had improved, which is great. Strikingly, there was no difference between the rates of improvement between the groups i.e. two yoga classes per week were as effective as a restrictive diet for improving symptoms in this common disorder.

The number of common foods that are excluded on the low FODMAPS diet can make it very difficult to stick to and enjoy, so the availability of yoga as an effective alternative intervention, with all the additional benefits associated with the practice, makes this a great choice for IBS sufferers and, frankly, everyone.

The modern yoga renaissance has led to an explosion in different types of yoga practice. From the detailed and precise Iyengar to the fast-flowing and demanding Rocket, there truly is something for everyone. I strongly suggest checking out local classes and giving them a go. There are also a great many classes available for free or with paid subscription online, making this a more accessible option for those with limited budgets. You may want to go to a few classes first to understand proper alignment before establishing a home practice, or doing a combination of the two.

Risk Factors

It is not all good news though. While regular PA confers numerous brain benefits across the lifespan, some sports carry significant brain risks that are important to understand.

Concussion, sub-concussion and post-concussion syndrome

A concussion is a form of traumatic brain injury that results from a blow to the head or the rapid movement of the neck, such as in a whiplash incident. While the symptoms (see opposite) may last for as little as a few hours or a couple of days, concussions pose a serious risk to long-term brain health.

While a helmet protects the skull from fractures, as you can see from the diagram below, the brain is not fixed or held in place within the skull. Rather it is suspended in (or cushioned by) a thin layer of cerebrospinal fluid. This means that when there is an impact or a rapid, forceful movement, the brain slides within the skull and is pressed against the hard inner skull walls. The brain is very soft and is easily damaged by these kinds of impacts, and research is showing us that the damage can be severe and long-lasting.

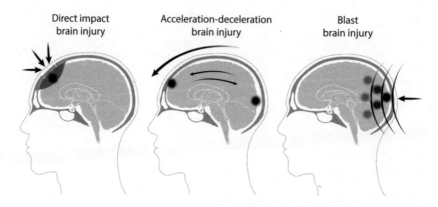

| Direct impact brain injury | Acceleration-deceleration brain injury | Blast brain injury |

What happens to the brain in a concussion? The brain experiences both structural and functional damage during a concussion:

- Axons are damaged, impairing or severing communication between brain cells.
- Cell membranes around the cell body (soma) are damaged. This can lead to the leaking out of ions into the intracellular space, where they can disrupt the function of other nearby cells.
- Cellular energy is depleted as cells work to repair the damage and the balance of compounds within the affected cell.
- Mitochondria, the powerhouse of the cell, are damaged or functionally impaired, creating an energy deficit in the cell, promoting negative cognitive symptoms.
- The impact may also cause blood vessels to break causing bruising (cerebral contusion).
- Inflammatory processes are upregulated in response to the injury.

Symptoms of a concussion
- dizziness
- confusion
- memory problems
- headaches
- tinnitus (ringing in the ears)
- nausea or vomiting
- visual problems such as 'seeing stars' or blurred vision
- irritability
- low mood or depression
- problems with balance
- loss of consciousness (though you can still be concussed without losing consciousness)

Subconcussion A subconcussive injury is one in which the damage to the brain is not severe enough to create obvious symptoms. However, there is growing evidence that repeated collisions that lead to subconcussive injuries cause diffuse damage to the brain, which only becomes apparent years after the injuries were acquired.

Post-concussion syndrome Around 15 per cent of people who experience a concussion will go on to develop post-concussion syndrome, in which they suffer many of the symptoms outlined above as well as impaired taste and smell, fatigue, anxiety, sleep disturbance and light sensitivity for days, weeks and sometimes months following the injury. These symptoms may be managed with a combination of medication and psychological therapy.

Chronic traumatic encephalopathy

For a couple of years I trained at a local boxing gym. My fitness was pretty good and my longs arms mean I have a decent reach, so my trainers would encourage me to do more sparring. But, try as I might, and as much as I enjoyed the sport, I could never settle into it. My sparring partners all told me the same thing, 'You think too much.' They were absolutely right. What I was thinking about was what happens to the brain when you take a blow to the head!

The brain, at the same time as being wonderful, is incredibly fragile. Its function can be affected by something as innocuous as losing a couple of hours' sleep, drinking a glass of wine or having negative thoughts. Still, every day healthy people expose this delicate organ to harm in the form of contact sports, and we are beginning to see the effects in startling rates of degenerative neurological disorders in former athletes.

Punch drunk, boxer's brain, dementia pugilistica ... These terms were coined in the 1920s to describe the neurological symptoms seen in former boxers, which included slurred speech, memory impairments, confusion and tremor, and were associated with the repeated concussions received during fights. But it is not only boxers who are exposed to these kinds of repetitive brain traumas. Dementia pugilistica is now known as chronic traumatic encephalopathy (CTE) and it was first identified in American Football players by neuropathologist Dr Bennet Omalu.

The image below shows the difference between a healthy human brain and one in the chronic stages of CTE:

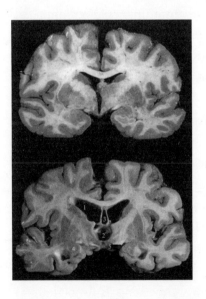

Gross pathology of CTE
Top: Coronal section of a normal human brain.
Bottom: Coronal section of a brain from a retired professional football player, showing the characteristic damage associated with CTE.

The thick hard shell of the skull is meant to protect the delicate brain from the occasional accidental impact. It is not designed to cushion repeated deliberate blows. When head traumas are repeated, even without concussion, the brain is unable to repair this damage; the brain is in a state of chronic inflammation.

In a 2017 review CTE was identified in 99 per cent of the brains of former National Football League (NFL) players. In a recent interview Dr Omalu said:

> No child under the age of 18 should be engaging in the high-contact sports: football, ice hockey, rugby, MMA, boxing, wrestling. One season results in permanent brain damage. If we wouldn't give a child a cigarette . . . why would we place a helmet on the head of child and send him into a field to intentionally smash his head against the heads of other children?

The NFL is currently being sued by former players for claims that the repeated head collisions and concussions received during their footballing careers contributed to their neurological disorders. As of May 2019 the NFL had paid out over $650 million in claims.

South Africa Rugby manages concussions in the game with the 'recognise and remove' process, which permits the referee to discharge from the game a player with an obvious or suspected concussion. Along with the familiar red and yellow penalty cards, referees can now issue blue concussion cards, immediately removing the athlete from play and initiating the process of neurological assessment and graduated return to play.

Informed consent

In any free society adults are free to participate in any legal leisure or sporting activity, even when those activities pose significant risks to long-term health or life. However, individuals can only be said to have had 'informed consent' if they were made aware of the risk at the outset. If you participate in any sport or activity that carries a reasonable risk of body slams or blows to the head you should be aware that you are at significantly increased risk of brain injury. These sports include:*

- American football
- BMX
- boxing
- football (heading the ball and accidental head collisions)
- ice hockey
- kickboxing
- mixed martial arts
- motocross
- roller derby
- rugby
- snowboarding
- wrestling

Dehydration

Exercising for long periods or at high intensities induces dehydration through sweating. The effects of acute dehydration on the body include: reduced blood volume (putting pressure on the heart); lowered testosterone; elevated cholesterol; disrupted electrolytes; and damage to the kidneys. But water is not only lost from muscles, it is lost from the whole body, including the brain. What effect does this water loss have on brain health?

* Outside of sport, it should be recognised that victims of domestic violence and individuals who self-harm by head-banging are also at risk of subconcussive and concussive injuries and should be monitored for cognitive symptoms.

Firstly, the brain shrinks and the more dehydrated the body is, the more the brain shrinks. This means there is more room in the skull for the brain to move. This is particularly relevant to contact sports that include a risk of blows to the head because, combined with the force of a blow, we can expect that there will be a more forceful impact, and consequently more damage.

Secondly, in a dehydrated state the brain has to work harder to carry out normal processes, resulting in increased tiredness and perceived effort.

Dehydration is a challenge for the brain and may be particularly detrimental for children and adolescents (neurologically, the brain is still developing into the mid-twenties).

Takeaways
- Next to sleep, regular physical activity is the best investment you can make to your long-term brain health.
- For the most part, PA is a powerful tonic for the brain, improving perfusion, function, plasticity and cognitive reserve, and reducing the risk of highly prevalent disorders such as depression, anxiety and Alzheimer's disease.
- We tend to think of movement as a bit of a chore. Try to think of all physical activity as an opportunity to improve the health of your brain.
- PA increases neurogenesis and can, in effect, reverse brain ageing.
- Exercise can help to mitigate the negative effects of chronic stress on the body by reducing the circulation of neurotoxic compounds in the bloodstream.
- People who participate in regular physical activity have better brain function and are more likely to retain their cognitive abilities as they age.

- All forms of activity count: aerobic, resistance training, HIIT and walking all infer brain, mood and mental health benefits. The emphasis is to simply move.
- There may be additional brain benefits to doing exercise that involves an element of learning or balance such as dancing or yoga.
- Contact sports (and any activity that incurs a likelihood of concussion) are associated with increased brain-health risks, even when helmets are worn.
- It is right that you (especially parents of children and adolescents) know that every blow to the head or concussion increases the risk of later developing cognitive impairment or CTE.

CHAPTER 10

Using the Breath

In the opening chapters I described how the balance of health and well-being can be thought of as the balance between healthy and unhealthy stress; too little of one and too much of the other impairs physical and psychological resilience. While good-quality sleep, a healthy diet and plenty of exercise will contribute to brain health and emotional well-being, it may not always be convenient to grab a quick nap, a snack or start doing lunges in the middle of that important meeting. However, there is one powerful, criminally underused tool that is always available to you: your breath.

No doubt, at some time in your life when you have been anxious or distressed, some well-intentioned person has instructed you to 'take a deep breath'. More than likely their suggestion felt rather glib but in this chapter I hope to convince you that it's much more than a tired cliché, an old wives' tale or esoteric mumbo jumbo. Properly utilised, your breath can significantly improve your emotional resilience and psychological performance in a given task.

How Controlled Breathing Can Reduce Depression

A fascinating series of trials provides evidence that a breathing intervention might be useful in the fight against the main cause of our looming mental health crisis: depression. In this randomised, single-blinded study 25 depressed patients, who had had limited improvement from antidepressant medication, were allocated to either participate in a breath-based meditation practice, called Sudarshan Kriya Yoga (SKY), or a waiting list for eight weeks. The participants on the waiting list acted as the control group in the study and were offered the meditation course at the end of the study period.

The breathing techniques were drawn from one of the core arms of yoga (pranayama) and included:

- Ujjayi breathing: a long, slow audible breath created by gently constricting the throat and breathing through the nose.
- Bhastrika: a rapid, 'pumping' nasal breath created by forcefully constricting the abdomen.
- Chanting of 'Om': an elongated note that creates vibration in the chest, throat, jaw and ears.
- Sudarshan Kriya: cyclical breathing, in which the practitioner alternates between closing one or other nostril.

All parts of the practice were completed sitting in a comfortable position with eyes closed. Participants were instructed to focus on the sensations within their bodies. During the initial week, participants practised SKY along with yoga and received information on the nature of stress. For the remainder of the eight weeks they were advised to practise SKY for 20–25 minutes per day at home and attend a 90-minute class once a week.

Levels of depression were assessed using the Hamilton Depression Rating Scale 17 (HDRS17), a well-established questionnaire in depression research that has 17 questions. The scoring on the HDRS17 is as follows:

- 0–7: normal range
- 8–16: mild depression
- 17–23: moderate depression
- >24: severe depression

At the start of the trial the participants had an average score of 22. For those who completed the programme (two people dropped out) the depression score dropped by 11.5 points – a dramatic change, especially when we consider that these were patients who had not responded to medication. In comparison, the mean score for those on the waiting list increased by 0.5 points.

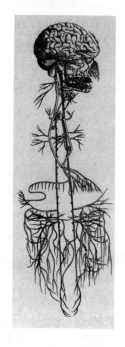

Separate trials of controlled breathing have shown that it significantly reduces anxiety and depression in male lung disease patients compared to controls, and cancer patients. Why might this be? In order to understand, we first need to meet the vagus nerve.

The vagus nerve

This multitasking nerve gets its name from the Latin for 'wandering', a reflection of its wide-reaching connections and effects across the body. As you can see from the image, the vagus nerve starts in the brain stem, runs through the throat and larynx (voice box), down into the chest, through the heart and lungs, and all the organs, including the liver and kidneys, before reaching the gut. Indeed, it is the main direct highway between the gut and the brain. If you think about it as a highway with 10 lanes, at least eight of the lanes would be going upwards, from the body to the brain (afferent nerves), rather than the reverse (efferent). In this way the vagus nerve is always relaying information about what is going on in the body back to the brain.

However, it would be wrong to think that the vagus is just a messenger. This nerve is the main structural component of the parasympathetic nervous system (PSNS), the part of our nervous system that is responsible for rest, relaxation and recovery, as well as regulating heart rate and respiration (see page 36).

The vagus nerve is potently anti-inflammatory. Stimulating the vagus nerve leads to the release of acetylcholine, which blocks the release of pro-inflammatory cytokines. Rats that were injected with harmful bacteria were saved from going into toxic shock by way of vagus nerve stimulation (see page 166). In humans, it shows promise as a safe and effective treatment for rheumatoid arthritis, a chronic inflammatory disease, even in patients who have shown a poor response to standard medications. A small trial of vagus nerve stimulation on Crohn's disease (intestinal inflammation) patients produced reduced symptoms and lower levels of inflammatory cytokines.

Does this anti-inflammatory effect mean that there is a role for the vagus nerve in the treatment of depression? Potentially. Vagus nerve stimulation is already approved as a treatment for epilepsy and depression by the American Food and Drug Administration.

In the UK, the National Institute for Health and Care Excellence has said that, as yet, there is insufficient evidence to support the widespread use of vagus nerve stimulation in treatment-resistant depression, but it may be used if the patient is made fully aware of the limitations or for research purposes. Further research is currently underway.

> **Vagus nerve stimulation**
> Medical stimulation of the vagus nerve involves surgery to implant a small pulse generator (like a pacemaker) under the collarbone of the patient. An electrode is coiled around one of the branches of the vagus nerve. The generator produces an electric pulse that stimulates the nerve. Side effects of vagus nerve stimulation, such as hoarseness, sore throat and headaches, tend to be mild and tolerable.

Where the vagus nerve passes down the neck, its activity can be influenced by breathing practices, with at least theoretical potential as a mental health intervention. This is understood to be the primary way that breathing can have antidepressant effects. The resistance created by constricting the throat muscles during controlled breathing activates the afferent fibres of the vagus nerve, which then produces biological responses consistent with its role in relaxation.

Magnetic resonance imaging (MRI) scanners produce detailed images of what is happening in the body and are used routinely in medicine to identify evidence of disease or the location of obstructions. An innovative study scanned the brains of 12 healthy volunteers as they chanted 'Om'. The scientists identified a pattern of widespread brain deactivation in the amygdala, the anterior cingulate and the hippocampus, areas associated with threat detection, emotion processing, memory, pain perception and stress reactivity, that they believe to be mediated by vagus nerve activation.

Singing

It's not just breathing; the vagus nerve is involved in the motor activity of the diaphragm, which means that any activity that stimulates diaphragmatic movement will activate the vagus nerve, including singing.

Singing has been linked to lower average blood pressure and reduced incidence of depression. People who are members of a choir also report greater feelings of resilience and an increased sense of social connectedness, all factors that are associated with better long-term mental health.

Nasal Breathing and Memory

Could there be a relationship between breathing and memory function?

If you recall from Chapter 3, the olfactory nerve (the one in the nose) has a direct connection to the frontal lobe, and particularly the hippocampus and the amygdala, which is why smells can quickly evoke powerful memories. However, it is not just smelling; the very mechanics of breathing through the nose appear to influence brain activity.

In a series of fascinating trials researchers were able to directly observe the electrical activity of the brain in response to different types of breathing. In the first part of the trial, researchers observed that electrical activity in certain areas of the brain synchronised with the pattern of nasal inhalation and exhalation. This pattern of activation started in the piriform cortex, the area associated with our sense of smell, but then spread to include the amygdala and the hippocampus. The researchers suggest that breathing in through the nose acts as a kind of regulator, synchronising electrical activity across the brain.

This activation and synchronicity also seems to influence cognition. In a later trial, 21 healthy participants were asked to view images of either surprised or fearful faces, and to judge whether the face was fearful or surprised as quickly as possible. All the while the research team monitored performance as the participants breathed in and out. What they found was truly remarkable: the recognition of fearful faces and the ability to accurately recall information was significantly better when the participants viewed the original image during a nasal inhalation.

In another experiment 75 healthy participants viewed a series of faces. Twenty minutes later they viewed another series of faces and were asked to identify which ones they had already seen. The people who had viewed the faces while they were breathing in through their noses accurately recalled more faces than those who viewed them while exhaling. This was a small trial but the results suggest that this nasal inhalation pattern of activation may improve information processing and cognitive performance.

The 4-4-8 breath

Most of us spend the majority of our time taking shallow breaths. Slow controlled breathing that fully engages the diaphragm and utilises the constriction of the throat (activating the vagus nerve) is an accessible way to promote calm. If you are not used to diaphragmatic breathing it can feel a little strange to start. This exercise should help.

- Lie comfortably on the floor (or your bed) with your knees bent and your feet on the floor.
- Place your hands on your belly so that the tips of your middle fingers meet at your belly button.
- To a slow count of four take an inhalation through your nose, drawing the air into your belly so that your fingertips are gently drawn away from each other. This can sometimes take a few goes, particularly if you are a habitual shallow breather.
- Hold the breath for another count of four.
- Breathe out through your nose, with control, for a count of eight. You will find that you need to slightly constrict the back of your throat to slow the exhalation.
- Continue for at least two minutes, repeating this four-four-eight pattern.

(To count the breaths think 'one elephant, two elephant . . .' Your count of four may be longer but not shorter than this. If you have respiratory or blood pressure issues, or feel dizzy when doing this exercise, please stop and return to breathing normally.)

The Downsides

Air pollution

Air quality is of increasing concern and there is growing scientific literature that shows that air pollution is a significant health risk, particularly for those living in urban areas or close to busy roads.

A new study raises specific concerns about the damage that chronic exposure to polluted air can inflict on our brains. Researchers looked at data from 162 areas of China, a country with some of the worst air quality in the world. The data compared levels of air pollution against scores on tests of cognitive abilities such as verbal skills and mathematics. They found that worse air quality was associated with worse cognitive performance. A paper published the year before, which tracked over 6 million Canadians, indicated that living near a busy road can increase a person's risk of being diagnosed with dementia by 12 per cent.

The protection of the still-developing brains of babies, children and adolescents should be a public health priority, with measures put in place for the improvement of air quality in areas where they congregate, such as nurseries, schools and playgrounds.

Smoking

Smoking is a kind of air pollution that smokers generate for themselves. Much is known about the harms of smoking on the body, but what about the brain? By now you should know that if something damages the body it will also harm brain health and this is absolutely the case with smoking. Cigarette and cigar smoke contains around 100 compounds that are known to be hazardous to health, and many that are toxic to brain cells such as carbon monoxide, aldehydes and cyanide. Cigarette smoke contains high levels of reactive oxygen species (see page 127), contributing to increased cellular oxidative stress.

The brains of smokers tend to be smaller, with thinner cortices, decreased blood flow and more areas of damage. Correspondingly, regular and long-term smokers have poorer brain function, scoring lower than non-smokers on tests of attention, language, planning, reasoning, memory, processing speed and cognitive flexibility. Smoking also increases an individual's risk of developing dementia, with some estimates suggesting that up to 14 per cent of global Alzheimer's cases are attributable to smoking.

Encouragingly, if a person is able to stop smoking there is evidence that some of the brain damage associated with smoking is reversible, but it takes several years. In short, if you are a smoker, the sooner you stop, the better.

Takeaways

- The way we breathe may influence brain activation, and controlled breathing practices have the potential to influence several biological systems, including cortisol, heart rate and even cognitive performance.
- The vagus nerve has a potent anti-inflammatory and regulatory effect on the body.
- Controlled breathing is the most accessible way of influencing the vagus nerve and activating the PSNS.
- Two minutes of slow nasal breathing has been shown to reduce symptoms of stress and depression. Try the 4-4-8 breath when you begin to get a rising feeling of stress or panic.
- Mindful movement practices, such as yoga, that combine controlled breathing with gentle movement are effective stress management interventions and valuable adjuncts to standard treatment.

- Singing offers multiple mechanisms for improving brain health including lower levels of stress hormones and reduced depression.
- Air pollution poses a risk to health including cognitive function. If you cycle in built-up areas be sure to use a protective mask. If you smoke, contact your local smoking cessation service to try to reduce or stop altogether.

CHAPTER 11

Understanding Emotions

Many people have the impression that emotions are at best incidental (they just crop up unannounced for no good reason) or at worst a nuisance (when they do pop up they just cause trouble). However, our emotions are not only involved in feeling states such as happiness or sadness; they also inform aspects of motivation, reward and meaning. Our emotions are *essential* for giving our decisions purpose and helping us to make choices in the direction of a goal. When you make decisions your brain cross-references information from the outside world (like what is useful and socially acceptable) with feedback from the internal world about what feels right, makes sense or is important for you.

In my clinical experience I have found that much of this misperception about emotions relates to a fundamental lack of understanding of the nature and function of emotions. A highly nuanced perception of our feeling states and the ability to represent and communicate those states through language are two features that distinguish us most from other social species. While other animals such as apes, cats and dogs seem to express states that we would recognise as fear, anger and affection, humans seem to be the only ones that have the capacity to reflect on those states and describe them to others. Rather than simply being a quirk of human life, this ability for emotional reflection is, I believe, absolutely crucial to our success as individuals and as a species. Emotions are also the language of relationships. Having the emotional skills to initiate and sustain healthy relationships is one of the strongest protective factors for long-term mental health and psychological resilience.

One of the great achievements of human civilisation is our extraordinary knack for collaboration; individuals come together to work on a shared goal. Imagine a past scene: a group of humans arrive on a new area of land. There is access to water, the land appears fertile and there are grazing animals nearby that would provide a reliable food source. This looks like a good place to inhabit. Now there is just the issue of shelter. In the absence of natural shelter (such as a cave formation) we would need to construct a suitable dwelling from the available materials. It would be hugely inefficient for each person or family to attempt to do this alone; there would be a high degree of failure, wasted materials and hunting time lost. A much better system is for members of the group to collaborate and work together to build each other's homes.

The same goes for other labour-intensive survival tasks, such as hunting, food preparation and child-rearing. So we learned how to live and work together as members of larger and larger communities. However, there is a trade-off to living as a group. We are also a deeply territorial and anxious species. Our evolutionary histories are defined by conflicts over land, possessions and reproductive opportunities (which happen to all be related). In order to survive and reproduce we had to be able to fight for what was ours, defend our own territory and, at times, annex the territory of our rivals.

For these evolutionary reasons some emotions, such as aggression, seem to be hardwired into us. Aggression is an innate social behaviour for which we require little if any teaching. Even small children can be seen to lash out with their fists when faced with a situation that is frightening or unfair. Neuroscientists have even managed to identify the seat of aggression in the mammalian brain. A tiny structure, composed of only around 10,000 neurones, in an area called the ventromedial hypothalamus, seems to be the brain circuit for aggressive behaviour. To demonstrate this, researchers insert an electrode into this area of a mouse or rat brain and when they stimulate it with an electric current they can cause an otherwise docile animal to attack a non-threatening roommate. So aggression has a fixed circuit in the brain. Can you see the problem? On the one hand we have an evolutionary drive to aggressively defend what we see as our property, whether that's physical, sexual or intellectual. On the other, we live in complex social communities on which we are deeply dependent on each other for the fulfilment of our survival needs and existential ambitions.

This is where emotional reflection comes in and why that deep connection between the cool, rational prefrontal cortex and the hot, instinctive limbic region is so beautiful. Emotional reflection allows us to critically appraise, understand and, where necessary, overcome our instinctual responses. Having the ability to take an objective look at what we are feeling, to make an attempt to understand the trigger for it and then, crucially, to describe this to someone else in the form of a negotiation is one of the most fundamental aspects of democracy and civilisation. It is the essence of diplomacy and the means with which we are able to reduce our reliance on our aggressive instincts.

Creating Emotionally Healthy Environments

The foundations for how we relate to our emotions as adults are laid in childhood. This raises the important question of how to promote healthy emotional functioning in children. In my profession it is often said that a parent's job is to help their child to leave them, which is to say that parents have a huge responsibility in helping to prepare their children for life as independent, resilient, compassionate adults. From my point of view, one of the most important tasks of parenting is to help the child to understand their emotional worlds. This is a multifaceted task that includes:

- Providing the child with the appropriate vocabulary to identify their emotional states.
- Creating a caring environment in which the child is safe to express the full range of emotions (including those that are often described as 'negative') without imposing unreasonable or age-inappropriate conditions on the child.
- Helping the child to de-escalate from intense emotional experiences.

When done consistently (which doesn't necessarily mean perfectly), in most cases the child will come to learn that:

- These powerful internal sensations can be understood and are nothing to be afraid of (this is crucial in helping to limit the distress of intense emotions).
- They are worthy of love for the total of who they are, not just the 'nice' aspects (this is the foundation of good self-esteem).
- Pain is temporary and they have the appropriate coping

mechanisms to recover from difficult events (this is the corner-stone of psychological resilience).

You can see how what a person learns about their emotions during childhood has profound effects on their mental well-being in adulthood. Psychologically, we talk about how responses to emotions can be validating or invalidating.

Emotionally invalidating environments

There are some characteristic ways of responding to others' emotions that have been demonstrated to be psychologically damaging. These 'emotionally invalidating environments' and the emotional inhibition they engender have been linked to the development of borderline personality disorder, increased risk of depression, anxiety disorder, post-traumatic stress disorder, obsessive compulsive disorder and impairments in one's sense of self. But what do these environments look like?

Emotionally invalidating environments are those in which the child receives the consistent message that their emotions are:

* wrong or inappropriate ('You're so dramatic')
* irrational, stupid or childish ('You're being overly sensitive. You're such a baby')
* unwelcome, 'too much' or a burden ('I can't deal with you right now')
* less relevant than the emotions of others ('How do you think I feel?')

In effect, the child's emotions are thrown back at them or they are left having to deal with them by themselves. However, this is no easy task because the emergence of a powerful or difficult emotion can be very frightening for a child or adolescent. Emotions are visceral – we may feel hot, sick or dizzy. We may find it hard to breathe and our hearts might start pounding in our chests. If you've ever had a moment of absolute terror or panic you can understand how all-consuming that emotional experience can be. Now imagine being a child and experiencing these things for the first time. Intense emotions can often be utterly overwhelming for the child's level of psychological maturity and this is why it is so important that a kind, thoughtful and aware adult is available to help them to navigate their way out of this new, important but challenging experience.

A range of responses to the child's feelings may constitute invalidation:

- sarcasm and minimising
- dismissal
- rejection
- denial
- guilt trips (e.g. 'I know you're sad but I need you to be happy for me otherwise I will be upset')
- stonewalling, silence or the cold-shoulder
- condescension and mockery
- comparisons to others' suffering ('It could be worse. You think you've got it bad . . .')
- conditional love ('I don't love you when you are like this' or behaviour to that effect)
- parental emotional dysregulation (when the parent becomes distressed when faced with the child's upset. Here the child learns that it is potentially dangerous to others for them to express their feelings)

The invalidator may be anyone whose opinion of the person matters: parents, friends, teachers, sports coaches, or partners in adulthood. When thinking developmentally (ages 0–16ish), the invalidating environment is usually created by parents or siblings.

One of the challenges that clients often come up against when thinking about how their developmental/family environment may have caused them harm is intentionality: 'They were doing their best and they would be so upset if they knew I felt like this.' One thing I try to impress upon my clients is that therapy is not about 'blame', rather it is about facing reality, and reality is often complex. People may behave in emotionally invalidating ways for any number of important reasons for which they too deserve compassion, such as:

- their own unprocessed trauma, anger or resentment
- emotional immaturity
- overwhelm
- unmanaged mental health issues
- alcohol or substance issues
- chronic stress

They may well have been trying their best in the circumstances. However, it is also true that, despite their best efforts, the reality is that the environment they created contributed to the transmission of psychological distress to the child and this too deserves compassion and recognition. Research evidence shows that the degree of parental emotion invalidation predicts emotional inhibition and socially avoidant behaviours in their children.

Now, it is worth saying that sometimes these attitudes leak out even in healthy relationships, and it is especially likely to happen when there is a high degree of external stress. However, it is again the case that the 'dose is the poison'; in healthy families invalidating interactions happen rarely and, ideally, there is reparation in the form of an appropriate apology. In emotionally invalidating environments the response is more likely to be undermining than validating.

It is also true that we may find ourselves in invalidating environments at any time of life. For example, we see it in action in unhealthy romantic relationships in adulthood, often as a form of control. However, it is particularly psychologically harmful during childhood as it has the effect of distorting the child's sense of reality long into adulthood, and can erode self-esteem.

Emotionally validating environments

In contrast, an emotionally validating environment is one in which one's psychological world is accepted, taken seriously and available for compassionate, non-defensive discussion. Emotionally validating statements might be:

- 'I understand that you are angry.'
- 'I can understand why you are upset.'
- 'I'd like to understand why you feel like this. Can you tell me what you're feeling?'
- 'Do you know why you feel like this? Do you think there are any causes?'
- 'I'm sorry that my [behaviour] hurt you.'

You may have noticed that these statements all focus on understanding the other person's experience and, where appropriate, taking responsibility for the impact of our actions on others' well-being. Similarly, it is important that we validate our own emotions. Instead of thinking of ourselves as 'stupid' or 'childish' for experiencing certain emotions, we can acknowledge that there are reasons for what we feel, and that emotions are a normal and essential part of life.

Many people worry about being weak or 'overly indulgent' by acknowledging their feelings. However, emotional validation, of ourselves and others, actually contributes to psychological resilience, speeding up how quickly we recover from emotional distress and strengthening our ability to build strong, healthy relationships, which are crucial for good mental health.

Understanding introversion

Introversion is a personality trait characterised by a greater focus on one's own internal and mental states. Introverts tend to prefer solo activities or interacting with small groups of people at a time. In contrast extroverts tend to enjoy interacting with larger groups of people, and more often. Introversion is often mistaken for shyness or aloofness but introverts may be perfectly comfortable and confident in their preferred type of company.

Most of us live in societies in which extroversion and being 'outgoing' is highly prized. This cultural attitude can leave introverts feeling inadequate or finding themselves forced to participate in activities that they do not enjoy. This can be very unpleasant and even stressful. In fact, in my clinical experience I have found that introverts who have public- or group-facing jobs have a higher risk of stress-related issues like IBS.

It is important to respect and value that we all have different personality traits and preferences for how we like to spend our time. Being an extrovert is not 'better' than being an introvert. Introverts should not feel compelled to change to fit in. Instead they should focus on maintaining the relationships and activities that bring them support and satisfaction. Furthermore, extroverts should be mindful to respect an introvert's preference for quiet.

Emotional Inhibition

In the hugely successful musical *The Book of Mormon* Elder McKinley teaches the young missionaries to 'turn it off', to switch off unsettling thoughts or painful emotions 'like a light switch'. While this advice makes for hilarious comedy, it is a terrible strategy for psychological well-being.

Emotional inhibition is the habitual pattern of responding to difficult emotions with deliberate attempts to suppress or avoid emotion-related thoughts, feelings or expressions. Some emotional suppression may be socially adaptive – not screaming at a colleague for a mistake on a document is considered professional behaviour and definitely makes for a more conducive working environment. However, much emotional suppression is not adaptive and hinders social interaction and our own emotional development.

Early in therapy it is very common for clients to meet their own resistance when it comes to expressing painful emotions. Often they have been told that showing their feelings is a sign of weakness. It is also likely that, as children, many of them made the sad discovery that their emotional needs were too much for their parents and resolved, consciously or unconsciously, to try to put their emotions aside. When these people get to therapy, they have often rationalised this emotional rejection as the 'logical' belief that 'there's no point in feeling sad'. They are, though, very wrong.

'There's no point in crying'

Many, many people struggle with the experience of crying. However, crying has several functions.

First of all, you have three types of tears:

1. Basal tears keep the eyes lubricated.
2. Reflex tears help to wash out irritants such as dust blown in by the wind.
3. Psychic tears – a strictly human evolutionary adaptation – specifically for expressing emotion.

Clinical psychologist, Ad Vingerhoets, further subdivides psychic tears into:

1. Attachment-related pain tears.
2. Empathic, compassionate pain tears.
3. Societal pain tears.
4. Sentimental or morally based tears.

So, no matter how you look at it, all tears do 'something', and crying appears to have biological and psychological effects on both the person crying and on others.*

Individual effects

Psychologically, allowing yourself to cry is about recognising a real emotional state, which is crucial for good mental health. We'll see later on that emotions are important signals that, once you understand them, can help you to make significant life decisions. If nothing else, we all need to be able to face reality. If you can't accept that you are sad, how can you address the causes of your sadness?

Curiously, there seems to be an emotional rebound effect of crying. In the immediate 20 minutes after crying, people do tend

---

* We may also shed tears of happiness or surprise, but since people do not tend to struggle expressing these emotions, we shall focus here on tears of sadness.

to feel worse. However, ask them again 90 minutes after a cry and not only do they report feeling better than they did immediately afterwards, their mood is higher than baseline. Why might this be? There are a few possibilities.

The action of crying, which typically includes deep breaths, may stimulate the parasympathetic nervous system (PSNS), promoting relaxation and recovery. Another intriguing hypothesis involves a compound called nerve growth factor (NGF). Like BDNF, NGF promotes the growth and survival of neurones. NGF is present in lacrimal (tear-producing) glands and, consequently, also in tears, where it helps to protect and repair the eye surface. However, researchers speculate that it may travel, via the trigeminal nerve, to the brain where it acts in a similar way to BDNF. While more research is required to clarify this association, it suggests that the act of crying could aid recovery from the stressful events or circumstances that triggered the tears in the first place.

Social effects

In a series of trials in which participants were asked to judge the emotion being depicted from pictures of people's faces shown with or without tears, the presence of tears conveyed sadness more strongly. Seeing someone cry typically elicits compassion and empathy, a desire to help and offer support (what we call 'approach behaviour'), and therefore can strengthen emotional and social bonds. When tears are a genuine reflection of real emotions, and when those around us can recognise that, they usually have an attachment-enhancing effect – tears act as a social signal. Psychologically, tears are as legitimate and valuable as laughter.

Beyond the potential positive effects associated with crying, actively inhibiting your emotions actually undermines well-being.

The ironic effect

Emotional suppression is like trying not to think of a pink elephant; it is conceptually impossible because the act of trying not to think of something requires additional awareness, attention and energy. In studies where people have been told to suppress their pain (when holding their hands in iced water or watching a distressing video for example), participants who suppressed their feelings had less endurance and were much more fatigued than people who were allowed to show their discomfort.

This is known as the 'ironic effect'. Suppressing your emotions is demanding; it's harder and, at the end, the feeling you were trying to avoid is still there. The real tragedy of this irony is that though these behaviours are used in the hope of reducing emotional distress, they have been shown to significantly *increase* vulnerability to depression, generalised anxiety disorder, phobias, post-traumatic stress disorder, obsessive compulsive disorder and somatic symptoms like back pain. Emotional suppression also influences our eating behaviour: suppression worsens mood, leading most people to overeat low-nutrient, high-energy foods.*

One striking finding really emphasises the harm of emotional suppression. In a study published in 2014, a group of researchers assessed the habitual coping strategies of 625 teenagers (aged 14–19) who presented to emergency services for medical or psychiatric support. The teenagers were screened for significant life events (like break-ups or the death of a friend), suicidal thoughts or attempts, depression and tendency to emotional suppression. The analysis revealed that emotional suppression was the mediating

---

* In people who already have a lower body weight the opposite is seen: emotional suppression leads them to eat less, which has important implications for restrictive eating disorders such as anorexia nervosa.

factor between an adverse life event and the risk of suicidal thoughts or acts. Trying to hide their feelings increased these teens' risk of suicide. This is salient to what we teach children, especially boys, about how to deal with emotional pain.

Finally, holding back tears has serious negative effects on the body. It increases levels of stress hormones, raises blood pressure, activates the 'fight or flight' response, and is linked to elevated levels of harmful inflammation. It has even been linked to a greater risk of early death.

Time and time again, the results are the same: suppressing your emotions *increases and prolongs distress*, worsens mood, inhibits recovery and makes you *less resilient*.

I understand that not everybody who suppresses their emotions does so deliberately. Often the person has been conditioned by their environment – whether family, school, significant adults (such as a sports coach) or a significant (but unhealthy) romantic partner. But if you recognise yourself in these descriptions, working towards unlearning these habits is likely to have positive effects on your well-being. One way to begin undoing an emotional suppression habit is to start a 'one line a day' diary. At the end of the day simply write one or two sentences about how you felt during the day or how you feel in that moment. I often use this kind of diary as an orientation practice, helping clients to start acknowledging their feelings and get better at recognising their emotional reactions. You don't have to take any action to start with, the first step is awareness. Once you start to increase your emotional awareness you can extend this daily practice by asking yourself, 'What did I want in that moment that did not happen?' Or, 'What could I have done to improve the situation at the time?' Over time you can experiment with speaking up when the event occurs. In this way you can begin to be more assertive in your relationships (which is linked with greater confidence and self-esteem) and reduce the physical and psychological stress associated with emotional suppression, thereby helping to protect your brain and mental health.

Autonomic arousal

If you have watched the finals of an athletics competition you may have noticed some interesting behaviours in the athletes: pacing, puffing their cheeks, shaking their hands, swaying from side to side, sometimes even slapping their faces. As they prepare for this important moment in their professional careers, these sportsmen and women are experiencing elevated levels of autonomic arousal, and these movements are attempts to manage or discharge this 'nervous energy'.

If you are not an athlete you may still have experienced something similar; people often pace the room when they are angry, or chatter or laugh when they are nervous.

Autonomic arousal describes a complex array of physiological activity involving the whole body (i.e. including the brain) that translates as a readiness to act: the visual system is on hyper-alert, the stress response is activated so that cortisol and adrenaline are flowing, you become intensely focused on one thing and find it difficult to engage with anything else and, in your body, you feel agitated.

Any demanding activity, physical or emotional, like asking someone out on a date or receiving negative feedback, will elicit this feeling of agitation and I think it is this agitation that people refer to when they describe emotional or social experiences as 'awkward'. Your capacity to tolerate, manage and healthily discharge this agitation will influence how likely you are to try to avoid these intense or demanding, but often important, experiences.

Understanding Difficult Emotions

The biggest obstacle most people have with addressing difficult or unpleasant emotions is the negative connotation of the emotion itself. There are a handful of emotions that people think of as 'bad' or as an indication of a failure of thinking or self-control. The consequence is that they will be inclined to suppress, deny or avoid these emotions in the hope that if they do not look at them the feelings will disappear. This is another misunderstanding about emotions: that ignoring them will make them go away. I very often have to break the news to clients that this is not how it works. In reality, it is the opposite: emotional avoidance is associated with increased psychological distress.

Before I can convince anyone that there is value in acknowledging and expressing their 'negative' feelings, it is first necessary to bust some myths about these much-misunderstood experiences.

Envy and jealousy

These two emotions have a terrible public image. Firstly, they are often conflated as the same thing when there are subtle but important differences between the two. Secondly, they are characterised as 'petty' and dangerous, perhaps the motive for some hurtful act of vengeance. However, it is crucial to recognise that there is a difference between the awareness of an emotion and behavioural acting out. More often than not it is one's inability to *tolerate* and think about a difficult emotion that leads to attempts to discharge it in a physical and negative way. If we can learn to identify what we are feeling, understand what it means and draw on healthy coping mechanisms we will be much less likely to do harm to ourselves and others.

The first thing to recognise is that, psychologically, envy and jealousy are considered to be completely normal emotions that are valuable parts of a healthy emotional world. Influential child psychoanalyst Melanie Klein described how tiny babies and infants are capable of experiencing these powerful feelings. These emotions are innate and that may be because they are a feature of our evolved attachment systems. Attachment Theory describes how we are programmed to form strong psychological and emotional bonds to others – initially our parents or caregivers, and later our romantic partners and friends. It is thought that we are driven to develop these bonds because they increase the likelihood of survival, and the security of these bonds in childhood (from as young as two years old) has been shown to predict academic and professional success, and emotional well-being in adulthood.

In relationships, the major difference between envy and jealousy is the number of people. Envy arises between two people and relates to a feeling of wanting what someone else has, whether that is a material possession or a personal quality. For example, I may envy someone's musical talents or their new car. In this way envy is linked to perceived threats to self-esteem, such as the thought that I might not be as successful or talented as another person.

Jealousy usually involves three (or more) people and describes the intense feelings that accompany the perceived risk or fear of losing, or being left out of, a relationship. I may feel jealous when my best friend starts hanging out with someone new. The crucial point here is that jealousy often relates to the threat of *loss or exclusion*. If my friend makes new friends, they may care less about me. My fear is that I will lose this important relationship.

At their core, both envy and jealousy correspond to a sense of vulnerability. Vulnerability is a hugely uncomfortable feeling that most people try to ignore or avoid. However, if we are unable to identify the threats to self-esteem that underlie these feelings, and tolerate the vulnerability associated with them, there is an increased risk that we will try to externalise the problem or diminish the other person.

	Unprocessed	Processed
Envy	My neighbour has a flashy new car. I wish I could afford that. It's really not fair. She doesn't even need it. Her old car was fine. She's so greedy.	My neighbour has a very nice new car. Man, that makes me feel like I'm not doing as well in comparison. Then again, we're completely different people. The fact that there are things that I want does not mean that I can't be happy for her. Good for her.
Jealousy	My mate is hanging out with the new guy at the office again. I don't know what he sees in him. The guy is a loser. Not even remotely funny.	My mate is hanging out with the new guy at the office again. I guess it's good that they get on, but I do feel a bit left out. Maybe I didn't realise how much his friendship means to me. I should make sure I organise a night out.

Anger

If anger were a sports team, I would be its biggest fan. I'm sure that sounds strange, but, again, anger suffers from a huge amount of misunderstanding and bad PR. Similar to envy and jealousy, people often confuse the emotional experience of anger with the physical act of violence, but they are not the same thing. More than that, anger can be a driving force for tremendous good. Rosa Parks was motivated by her anger at the indignity of being told to sit at the back of the bus in 1950s racially segregated America. Her refusal to give up her seat was an act of defiance borne of righteous anger. And she helped to change the lives of millions.

Yet, we speak colloquially with disdain about anger, seeing it as a sign of immaturity or a lack of control. This mischaracterisation means that I sit with clients who have been stifling their legitimate anger for years and sometimes decades. Instead of acknowledging the anger, people will present to their GP or therapist with depression, anxiety, a physical symptom, or a drinking problem. So what lies at the root of anger and why should we be paying attention?

One hundred years ago Sigmund Freud outlined a theory of human psychology, one facet of which was the conflict between the two 'drives': life (sex) and death (aggression). It was Freud's observation that much of human mental life was played out somewhere along this continuum. Now, there is much for which it is easy to critique Freud but, in this particular case, I believe he is overdue some credit.

Neuroscientists from as far back as the 1940s isolated an area in the mammalian brain called the ventromedial hypothalamus (VMH), that when stimulated with an electrode elicits attack behaviour in an otherwise docile animal. More recently, Dr Dayu Lin, Associate Professor in the Department of Psychiatry at NYU, and her research team have demonstrated (in mice) that this area of the brain is also responsible for the generation of lordosis: the arching of the back that indicates that the animal is sexually receptive. So there is one key area in the brain in which sexual and aggressive behaviour is hardwired, providing a potential biological basis for Freud's observation. I should clarify that I am not saying that simply because an attribute is 'natural' that it is 'good', but appreciating that feelings of anger are as 'pre-installed' in the brain as sexual arousal should go some way to dispelling the myth that feeling angry is simply a sign that one is experiencing a lack of control.

Let's go further: there appears to be an interaction between the VMH and the dopaminergic (reward) system in the brain – there seems to be something *rewarding* about aggression. So, aggression appears to be *hardwired* into our brains *and* it is rewarding. Why might this be? As described earlier, the rewarding of aggression makes sense from an evolutionary perspective: an individual who could mount an aggressive response would be more effective at defending him/herself from attack and protecting their territory. In short, aggression is important for our survival, it forms part of our self-defence strategy. What does this tell us about anger in the modern world? We can take a clue from Ms Parks' actions. Anger is a signifier of injustice. Anger tells us that something in the world, or in the way that we are being treated, feels unfair, and this is what makes it so important that we do not ignore anger when it emerges. We should not ignore it but should we always act on it? This is the point at which we must engage the area of the brain that makes us uniquely human – the prefrontal cortex (PFC). After recognising feelings of anger it is incumbent upon us as wannabe rational beings to evaluate the *appropriateness* of the feeling in the current context, and then to adopt a suitable response.

For example, you are driving along and someone cuts in in front of you. Or you're standing in a long queue and someone decides that they don't need to wait in line like everyone else, and just inserts themselves in somewhere near the front. Most people would feel angry at this behaviour. Why? Because it's *unfair* that you are waiting and this person chooses not to. It's unfair that they are breaking the agreed social rules when others are keeping them. Now your response to this anger is a different story and this is where people trip up with thinking that the problem is the anger rather than the response to it. Some people might just tut, some might say something. In the worst situations, of course, this kind of behaviour can lead to road rage or physical violence. But again, this is the behaviour not the emotion, and the more we can understand and tolerate our feelings the more able we become at selecting the appropriate response.

Anger lite

It is indeed a bit of a cliché to say that therapists are obsessed with their clients being angry. However, the stigma and misunderstanding around anger often makes people, especially women, reluctant to ascribe this emotion to themselves. Instead, I listen out for any mention of the following descriptions – what I sometimes jokingly refer to as 'anger lite' – to give a clue as to whether what they are experiencing is in fact unacknowledged anger:

Aggravation	Envy
Agitation	Exasperation
Annoyance	Frustration
Aversion	Hostility
Boredom	Irritation
Disdain	Jealousy
Disgust	Resentment

Guilt and shame

Guilt and shame are another two emotions that are often mistaken for one another and that most people find very difficult to tolerate. While there is some overlap, there are important differences between how the two emotions are experienced and the behavioural responses they elicit. A very general way to distinguish between them is:

Guilt = *doing* wrong
Shame = *being* wrong

The sense of 'wrongness' makes guilt and shame deeply moral emotions linked to our place in society; guilt with a feeling that we have harmed another, shame conveying a belief that something about ourselves or our actions is inadequate. Behaviourally, shame is associated with social withdrawal and denial. Guilt tends to lead people to try to repair the damage that they feel they have done to another person.

The ubiquity of these emotions across diverse populations strongly suggests that they served an important purpose in our evolutionary past. Humans, particularly those in small subsistence tribes, depend on each other for survival, and an important feature of harmonious and productive coexistence is reciprocity – the principle of having a favour returned. However, without any penalties in place for wrongdoing it would be easy for an unscrupulous individual to play the system, to take without giving back. Such behaviour would benefit the individual (for a while) but do net harm to the group. Guilt and shame seem to be in-built psychological penalties for self-directed behaviours that might harm the overall well-being of the group.

A trial of 900 individuals from 15 small tribal communities across the world found a strong relationship between the amount of shame an individual felt when they imagined committing a misdeed and the degree to which the rest of the group devalued the action. That is to say that the intensity of shame felt predicted the actual degree of group disapproval. This relationship was seen in all the groups. The researchers argue that shame developed as an inbuilt mechanism to protect other people's opinions, and willingness to help us.

However, in modern, Western culture, it is true that many people experience excessive shame for attributes and activities unrelated to the welfare or well-being of society. Clients will often report feeling guilty about having a mean thought about someone or being ashamed of their body. When they are excessive and/or misplaced, guilt and shame can provoke harmful self-punishing behaviours, which can sometimes drive a further downward spiral of more guilt, more shame and worse punishment. I have also met people who have what is termed an 'unconscious' sense of guilt, in which the individual behaves as though they have done wrong, or are deserving of punishment but where no objective source of the feeling can be identified.

As with all of our emotions, it is important to interrogate what we are feeling and what it means. If your find yourself frequently experiencing intense feelings of shame and guilt the following questions can help you get to the root of the feeling:

- Am I feeling guilt or shame?
- If I'm feeling guilty, who do I feel I have wronged?
- Would that person agree that I have wronged them?
- If I told this story to a stranger would they agree?
- If I have truly hurt someone, how can I repair the relationship or make amends? (You may find 'How to Have Difficult Conversations' (on the next page) useful here.)
- If I am feeling shame, what do I think is wrong?
- Where did I learn that this aspect of me was bad?
- If a stranger told me they were feeling these things what would I say to them?

Of course, there is a tremendous amount of complexity and nuance involved in working through shame and guilt. If you really find it difficult to balance these emotions, it's important to seek professional support.

How to Have Difficult Conversations

One of the keys to living a fully engaged, authentic life is to learn the art of having difficult conversations. So many of life's most important problems can only be solved by summoning the courage to have a difficult conversation. Yet, for something that on the surface appears to be very straightforward, having 'The Big Conversation' is always a frightening prospect. I've seen corporate CEOs shudder at the idea of asking their parents to respect their decisions, for example. No matter who you are, or how successful you are in other parts of your life, there will be at least one big conversation that you're avoiding having.

Some examples of big conversations we often avoid
- Talking to a partner about sex.
- Talking to a partner about money worries or secret debts.
- Admitting that you are unsure about having children when your partner is keen to start a family.
- Telling a friend you have been hurt by their actions.
- Telling a parent you have felt unloved or rejected by them.
- Talking to children about sex, sexuality or sexual development.
- Disclosing that you are unhappy in a relationship.
- Having any conversation that might involve disagreement.

Here's why you shouldn't avoid an important conversation:

- The longer you put it off, the harder it will be.
- The longer you avoid it the more days of your life you live compromising your integrity by not being honest about your thoughts, feelings or who you are.

- Even if the other person can't understand or won't change, there is often tremendous value in demonstrating *to yourself* that you are worth sticking up for.
- You are massively underestimating the pressure that avoiding this conversation is putting you under. Every time you think about that person, the relationship or the event it chips away at your well-being and your emotional freedom to think about other things. If you can get the conversation out of the way, you free yourself of that burden.
- It builds emotional competence. Having one big conversation makes it easier to have another one. People who can speak honestly about their feelings benefit from having richer, more fulfilling relationships.
- It almost never goes as badly as you think it will. I say this as someone who has supported dozens of clients through what they thought would be the worst event of their lives. All survived and all said they felt much better for it.

Caveats

I think the big conversation is important to address but only if it is *safe* to do so. There are some conditions, emotional or situational, in which your well-being might be compromised by having it:

- If you rely on this person/people for emotional or practical support, and the cessation of that care would be deleterious for you.
- If there is genuine risk that you could be harmed by the discussion i.e. the other party has a history of violence. In this case it will be best to speak to a professional about other ways to manage this relationship.

- The big conversation should probably be avoided by people with a reliance on alcohol. In my experience, people often turn to drink in order to numb arousal i.e. to 'relax' or to shut down thinking. If this is the case, attempting an emotionally difficult conversation poses a risk of binge drinking. In this situation it is advisable to try to address the drinking and develop healthy emotional coping skills first.

In order to have this conversation, which is likely to elicit some anxiety, you must be familiar with tolerating the physiological agitation that comes with autonomic arousal (see page 187).

Bearing in mind that emotions are in large part physical experiences, I recommend that people develop a range of physical habits and practices to help them process and manage strong emotions, such as:

- walking (especially in nature)
- yoga
- dance
- a breath practice
- singing

How to do it

1. Remind yourself of the costs of the status quo. Make a list of all the ways that avoiding this conversation is diminishing your well-being: the awkward silences; the white lies; the anxiety; the suppressed anger. All of this compromises your physical and psychological health.
    Question: What is this avoidance costing me?
2. List all the ways in which you will benefit from having the conversation: greater confidence; more self-respect; improved resilience.

It's not just about this one conversation; these skills generalise so that you will feel more competent in other areas of your life. Question: How will I be better off in the long run if I can find the courage to do this?

3. Decide whether the benefits outweigh your fear and the risks. If so, you owe it to yourself to try.
   Question: Is it worth it?

4. Tell someone you trust that you are going to have the conversation. They can offer objectivity and support. Both are valuable. Of course, a therapist will be able to help you too.
   Question: Who can help me handle this?

5. Initiate the conversation. The toughest part is the start. Fortunately, modern technology provides us with several ways of laying the groundwork for a conversation. You can send someone a text or message asking when they would be free to talk. Once you have overcome this hurdle it should feel easier to actually say the words.
   Question: Can we make time to talk?

6. Prepare. Anxiety shuts down thinking so it is wise to prepare for how anxious you will be when you come to have the conversation. You may want to write some notes about what you would like to say. Sometimes people like to write a letter that they then read to the other person as it gives them a chance to thoroughly think through everything they want to say in advance. They can also then leave the letter with the other person to reread later.
   Question: What exactly do I want to say?

7. Do it face-to-face if you can. The reason that human faces are so expressive is because the subtleties of emotion expressed in the face are incredibly important in human

communication and social life. It is important that you make the most of the communication channels available to you.

Question: How can I make sure I do this properly?

8. Allow the other person time to think and respond. The other person may not have known that you felt this way or they may feel overwhelmed by emotions themselves. As much as you may want answers or explanations, it is fair to accommodate them. Be curious about their point of view.

   Question: How do they feel about it?

9. Leave time to recover. Remember: emotions take a physical toll on the body and this is likely to be an intensely emotional conversation. Don't plan to do anything afterwards. Clear your diary and make room for activities that will help reduce your levels of physiological arousal, such as walking through nature, journalling, or perhaps just sleep.

   Question: How can I reduce my physiological stress right now?

10. Plan for a follow-up. These conversations can be highly emotionally demanding, and it is not uncommon to miss things the first time round or for other thoughts and questions to emerge afterwards. Try to agree some space to address these additional issues.

    Question: Would it be all right if we have another conversation in a week or so, in case anything else comes up?

Everyday Emotion Management

In addition to being proactive in establishing practices that can reduce the risk of psychological decline, such as safeguarding your sleep, engaging in regular physical activity and addressing stress as soon as possible, I recommend making regular time to acknowl-edge your emotions. This need not be an arduous task. Perhaps a one line diary where you write, 'I felt nervous talking to my sister today. Still annoyed with her about what happened at the party.' This short practice promotes a mindset of emotional awareness and a greater sensitivity to when one's emotional health might be at risk of decline.

It can also be helpful to get into the habit of anticipating emotionally demanding situations. This can be achieved with a weekly 'start the week' practice where you write out and answer the following questions:

- How am I feeling about the week ahead?
- Which parts of my week are likely to be stressful or difficult?
- What can I do to prepare for these difficulties?
- If I do get stressed or overwhelmed what can I do to make myself feel better?
- Who can I tell that I am worried about this?

Why writing works
Like exercise for depression, writing as a means of managing emotions has become something of a cliché, which is a shame because it is a highly effective intervention, particularly for people who have a tendency for emotional suppression. First, it offers a means of low-threat emotional expression – you can release and reflect on your feelings without the risk of feeling judged. Secondly, in order to write about an emotion you have to think about it. This process renders something that feels vague and amorphous (feel-ings) into objects (words) that can be considered. In doing so, it becomes much easier to organise your thoughts, memories and

feelings into a coherent narrative, thereby transforming something that feels overwhelming into a neater, more manageable experience. Finally, going through this private reflective process can make it easier to talk to others – friends or a therapist – which is where recovery and growth accelerate.

Takeaways

- Emotional health *is* mental health. You cannot be psychologically resilient without an effective way to understand and manage your emotions.
- Emotions are highly evolved physiological sensations, many of which are hardwired into our brains.
- Emotional expression is a crucial part of interpersonal communication, relationships with others and personal well-being.
- Habitually suppressing your feelings is a form of chronic stress. Emotional suppression is not only ineffective, but is associated with greater risk of psychological and physical illness.
- The function of the PFC is suppressed under conditions of physiological or psychological stress. This means that we are less able to select an appropriate response to a strong emotion when we are stressed, and are more likely to act out in ways that we may later regret. Following the principles of basic self-care can help reduce the likelihood of this happening.
- Daily management of your emotional health should include both emotional and physical practices.
- So many of life's most important problems can only be solved by conjuring the courage to have a difficult conversation. Make a decision about whether it is worth the risk and safe to do so and, if the answer is 'yes', consider giving it a go.

- Expressive writing is an evidence-based intervention for emotional management. Making regular time to appraise the emotions and events of the day will increase general emotional awareness and your ability to respond appropriately to any challenges that emerge.

CHAPTER 12

Building
Psychological Resilience

One of the universal truths of life is that some pain is inevitable. There isn't one of us that gets through an entire human existence without experiencing some psychological or emotional distress. The timing of those events is important; we know that adverse events in childhood can create lasting mental health risks as those children move into adulthood. However, not every child or adult who experiences a painful or traumatic event will go on to develop a psychological illness. Resilience research looks at the aspects of someone's psychology that allow them to 'bounce back' from difficulty. Understanding these resilience factors has become an important part of mental health research and practice. Being able to identify those who are at higher risk will help us to better target treatments and might eventually allow us to coach at-risk individuals in the practices that build resilience, potentially preventing psychological illness.

One note of caution, though: we should be careful when talking about resilience that we do not infer that someone who develops a psychological illness is somehow 'weak' or 'not strong enough'. First of all, only a relatively small amount of our physical and mental health risk is in our hands (see page 309 for an explanation of why so much of our health is out of our individual control). Secondly, this means that most people who stay healthy managed to get lucky in some way: inheriting the right genes for their environment; avoiding hardship in childhood; having brain wiring that could tolerate the environment they found themselves in; having loving parents who supported their emotional and personality development, and so on.

Psychologists have identified a range of psychosocial habits and environmental factors that are linked to greater tendency to resilience in the face of trauma. In childhood these include:

- Good social skills
- Personal awareness of strengths and limitations
- Having empathy for others
- Warm and supportive parents
- Values social role, such as volunteering
- Extra-curricular activities

While some of these factors are down to fate, the majority are related to the child's psychosocial skills and the quality of relationships with parents and trusted others. Parents and adult carers can help to foster resilience in children by supporting them in understanding and expressing their emotions, encouraging them to work through difficulties with friends and engaging in team activities, in which children will be exposed to loss and failure, learning important lessons in how to manage these uncomfortable experiences.

In addition, psychiatrists Steven Southwick and Dennis Charney have identified a range of resilience-building factors that apply to both adults and children:

Social support

From the moment of birth, we are primed to build relationships. This is not an exaggeration; evolution has shaped babies' brains so that they can start to form relationships immediately:

- Although they will not have the muscular control to be able to focus their eyes until they are around two months old, babies prefer (i.e. pay more attention to) faces than any other objects in their visual field.
- Similarly, they pay greater attention to human voices than to other sounds.
- They show distress at being left alone, even when their other physiological needs have been taken care of.

Humans are social organisms; we are born into social networks and both our individual success and collective progress depends on our capacity to work together. Some of our most powerful emotions – those with the ability to alter our behaviour, such as guilt and shame – are indelibly linked to our relationships to other people and their opinion of us. And when it comes to resilience, the evidence is clear: we are stronger together.

We all benefit from having strong and supportive social relationships. In practical terms, that means someone who you feel close enough to to call in the middle of the night in an emergency, but also extends to feeling you have meaningful connections to family, neighbours and members of the wider community.

People with low social support have higher reactivity to stress, increased blood pressure, elevated heart rate and secretion of stress hormones – all factors that undermine brain health and resilience. In a trial of over 2,000 adolescents, friendship support was the greatest predictor of resilience. Having good social support has been shown to downregulate many of the inflammatory processes that are characteristic of the stress response, particularly in relation to chronic stress. People with good social support are also more likely to use healthy coping mechanisms when they experience adversity, which reduces the risk of creating additional negative outcomes.

It is one of the side effects of our busy modern lives that friendships can end up being neglected as we juggle work, family and romantic relationships. However, most people do not realise that our relationships are the major contributing factor to quality of life, above work and income. Having people on whom you can rely improves your physical and psychological health and enhances the meaning and enjoyment of life.

What I am saying is that most of us would benefit from a reassessment of our priorities when it comes to our relationships. Make a point of checking in with friends. Put it in your diary if you have to. Agree to a minimum of a monthly in-person catch-up to help maintain the quality of those bonds. Look for activity groups in your local community that you could participate in, whether that's walking, poetry or stand-up comedy. Do what you can to repair relationships that have been damaged or neglected (see 'How to Have Difficult Conversations', page 196). Investing in your relationships will enhance your well-being and your physical and mental health now and into the future.

Taking reasonable risks

In their book, *The Coddling of the American Mind: How Good Intentions and Bad Ideas are Setting up a Generation for Failure*, psychologist and lawyer Jonathan Haidt and Greg Lukianoff make the case that the soaring rates of psychological illness in people born after 1995 is in part associated with the limited opportunities these young people had to take manageable, age-appropriate risks during development. We saw earlier how vaccination entrains biological immunity by exposing the immune system to a weak version of a more dangerous disease. This enables the immune system to 'learn' how to identify and manage similar threats that it encounters in the future. A similar concept helps us to manage emotional distress and it is appropriately called 'stress inoculation'.

Stress inoculation involves giving yourself (or a child) the opportunity to grapple with a 'safe version' of a psychological or emotional risk in order to learn how to manage more complicated and significant situations in the future. For example, allowing children to fall out and make up while inventing games in the playground, without a parent or teacher swooping in to manage the situation, helps children to develop important interpersonal skills around turn-taking, conflict resolution and assertiveness. Children who are denied these opportunities (by well-meaning but overzealous parents or school admin policies) have fewer chances to develop these skills and, in later years, may find themselves overwhelmed in interactions with roommates at university or colleagues at work, for example.

Team sports and participation in competition are valuable environments for practising stress management and developing resilience. In team sports individuals must learn to cooperate and communicate effectively with others. Competition also provides important opportunities to learn how to fail.

Having a moral compass

It can seem a little old-fashioned to be talking about morality and values, but these concepts play a central role in understanding who we are, and having a clear sense of self-identity makes it easier to navigate difficult and ambiguous life challenges.

Having a clear set of moral values also eases the burden of decision-making and can help you feel more secure in the decisions you do make. For example:

Asher is ambitious and talented and has just been offered a well-paid position at a prestigious corporate firm. At the same time, Asher has always wanted to travel and an opportunity has opened up working for an international charity. Which should Asher choose?

On the face of it, this is a difficult decision, but if Asher is clear on her values, on what is intrinsically important to her, the decision becomes much easier. If what matters most is financial security, prestige and the kind of achievement available in the corporate world, she should take the job at the firm. If Asher most values travel, meeting new people and service, then working for the NGO is the clear favourite. Even if Asher later has doubts, there will be some consolation in the fact that, at the time, she made the decision that was most in line with her values and the kind of person she most wanted to be.

Having a moral compass helps us to feel that we are decent people and this fosters resilience because it reduces the tendency to self-punishment. For example, if something bad happens to me but I think I am a good person, I can be upset that it feels unfair but my self-esteem remains intact. Conversely, if something bad happens and I feel I am a bad or unworthy person, I am more likely to view this bad thing as my punishment for being a terrible human. Feeling that the whole world is against me would be damaging to my self-esteem and to my resilience.

A moral compass gives you grounding – a secure base from which to engage with the world.

Drawing on faith

Similarly, having a religious or spiritual faith has frequently been linked to improved well-being and even a longer life. This effect is not thought to be associated to belief itself, but to the habits and practices that are often enshrined in religious doctrine. For example, many faiths and spiritual practices encourage: compassion for others, service or volunteering, meditation or mindfulness, restrictions on alcohol and drug use and on extra-marital sex, and dietary limitations. These rules reduce an individuals' exposure to potentially harmful infections or lifestyle habits.

Regular group worship inculcates a community of individuals with a similar set of values who can be called on for advice or support in times of need. Loneliness has been identified as a major brain-health risk, with people who identify as lonely having a 40 per cent higher chance of developing dementia. The experience of belonging that comes with being part of a community is vital to our emotional well-being, reducing loneliness and the stress that comes with it.

Religious faith also provides believers with a reason for their existence and a sense of meaning in their lives. Having a sense of life purpose is independently associated with greater resilience (see page 214).

People who are not religious may benefit from emulating some of the core features of a religious lifestyle that are associated with improved well-being, such as regular face-to-face connection with friends, volunteering or some form of community service, regular quiet introspection and leading a purpose-guided life.

Good role models

To paraphrase John C. Maxwell: 'You will rise and fall to meet your expectations of yourself.' This is where values and role models become so important.

Individual executive control – the capacity to think about the consequences of an action and to work towards a stated goal – is influenced by peer expectation and affiliation. For example, in the Marshmallow Test, a classic experimental paradigm for testing delayed gratification in which children are rewarded with a second marshmallow if they can resist eating the first one for a few minutes, children who were told that they were a member of the group that waited for the second marshmallow were more likely to wait themselves. In everyday terms this translates to 'you are the company that you keep'.

A good role model is someone in whom we can partly identify. That means that we need to be able to recognise an aspect of ourselves or our life experience in this person. That might mean someone who grew up in our neighbourhood, had a similar upbringing or difficulties as us, has our skin tone, etc. Only if we can identify with someone whom we admire can we begin to conceive that we are capable of similar success (in whatever way that is defined for you). This fact forms the basis of why representation matters, or to put it another way, 'You cannot be what you cannot see.'

Seek out examples of people, similar to you, who are succeeding in a way that you admire or aspire to.

Being physically fit

As well as the brain health, emotional and stress management benefits of exercise, the same biological processes outlined in Chapter 9 contribute to psychological resilience. People who are physically fit express less physiological reactivity (lower heart rate, blood pressure and stress hormones) when they are exposed to a stressful life event. The hormetic adaptation to physical stressors also protects the mind when exposed to psychological stresses.

On top of this, the psychological habits required to attain and sustain physical fitness – such as persistence, distress tolerance, optimism, focus and impulse control – all contribute to better emotional health. Participating in group fitness also provides the opportunity to meet people and strengthen social support. Physical activity really is an incredible tonic for your mind.

Challenging your brain

Challenging your brain to learn new skills or to navigate novel environments supports neurogenesis, contributing to cognitive reserve, as outlined in Chapter 13.

Cognitive and emotional flexibility

'If all you have is a hammer, everything looks like a nail.' Cognitive and emotional flexibility is the art of applying the appropriate psychological response to the current circumstances, rather than over-relying on the same set of behavioural responses. Let's say you are a manager at work. Though you may consult your team, ultimately it will be up to you to make the final decision on the course of action to take. Your team will defer to you and ask for your sign-off on projects. However, it would be inappropriate to apply the same authoritative managerial attitude to your romantic relationship, where assuming superiority to your partner is likely to eventually result in resentment. Instead, in your relationship it makes more sense to work on communication, vulnerability and compromise in a way that might not be feasible in the workplace.

A flexible approach may sound obvious, but in reality many people struggle to achieve this level of adaptability. When we are stressed or sleep-deprived, functional connectivity between the prefrontal cortex (PFC) and the emotional processing centre of the brain is impaired and we are much more likely to revert to type: to apply one emotional response to all situations. This default position tends to be a cautious, anxious state. From an evolutionary perspective this fits – when cognitive resources are low it makes sense to err on the side of caution, to anticipate hostility or to assume everyone is a potential threat. However, in our modern lives, this approach more often than not simply undermines our sense of well-being and the quality of our relationships, making it more difficult for us to practise self-compassion or to ask for help.

Tips for building cognitive flexibility
- Find novelty. Try a new class, especially in something you have no interest in (you might be surprised by what you learn). Watch an online lecture on Greek mythology. Try a new cuisine. Try a physical challenge, like learning how to knit or running 5km. Visit a new town or city. Pushing yourself to do something unfamiliar can shift your thinking.
- Disagree with yourself. Take a subject that you feel very strongly about. This might be something like political beliefs

or abortion law, for example. Now, write a convincing argument, a paragraph or so, that completely disagrees with your original position. You will need to review other similar arguments to do this, which will push you out of your habitual way of thinking.

- Many paths to success. When faced with a problem, rather than thinking about *the* best solution, try to come up with three or four different ones. This can help to foster more creative and less narrow thinking.

Having meaning, purpose and growth in life

Viktor Frankl was a Jewish psychiatrist who was interned in the Nazi labour camps during the Second World War. In *Man's Search for Meaning*, written after his liberation, he describes his observation of the difference between the men who seemed more likely to survive the atrocious conditions they all suffered. He remarked that the prisoners who had defined for themselves a reason for living seemed able to draw on hidden reserves. Anecdotally, we often hear stories of elderly couples dying soon after each other. It is typically suggested that the second partner 'died of a broken heart'. This is a compelling narrative, but does it stand up to evidence?

In a startling example of the power of a purpose for life, psychologist Dr John Leach describes the characteristics of a phenomena called 'psychogenic death': 'people who respond to traumatic stress by developing extreme apathy, give up hope, relinquish the will to live and die, despite no obvious organic cause'. Dr Leach describes five stages of psychogenic death (colloquially known as 'give-up-itis'):

1. Social withdrawal, associated with a decline in mood.
2. Overwhelming apathy – total loss of motivation.
3. Aboulia – total loss of will or capacity to take decisive action.
4. Psychic akinesia – loss of connection to the body, including the perception of hunger and thirst, inability to make voluntary movements.
5. False recovery – a brief period where the person seems to recover some of these lost capacities. This recovery is short-lived, though, and the person soon dies.

Though the loss of a sense of meaning is rarely this dramatic, empirically, having a sense of purpose for our lives is associated with greater longevity, more years of healthy life, higher income and net worth, less use of health services, better engagement with preventative healthcare and better mental health.

So having a goal in life should not be considered a luxury – feeling that your daily activities have meaning contributes to better physical health and mental well-being. Sadly, most people underinvest in this aspect of their lives, perhaps because they believe that a sense of purpose is something that can only be achieved after reaching a certain level of financial success or social status. However, this is incorrect and it actually works the other way round: defining a purpose in life and working towards that imbues your life with more satisfaction, making the hard work required for success (however you define it) more intrinsically rewarding.

Ikigai

The Japanese concept of ikigai is a useful framework for defining the kind of work that will contribute to a purpose-driven life. Finding your ikigai requires outlining the activities that you love, are good at, that the world needs and that you can be paid for. The opportunity that fulfils all of these conditions is likely to be the one that provides you with a sense of meaning and a compelling reason to get up in the morning. I feel very fortunate that my job is one that fulfils all of these criteria for me, but of course not everyone wants to be a psychologist so your ikigai is unique to you.

To find your ikigai take a sheet of paper and sketch out the table below:

What I love	What I am good at	What the world needs	What I can be paid for

Hopefully there will be activities that appear in more than one column. Usually people are good at what they love (and vice versa). In this case the task is to identify an audience that will be willing to pay you for this. The Internet opens up a world of opportunities for previously impossible occupations – people will pay to watch other people play video games, for example. If you love playing video games and you're good at it this would be a great avenue to explore.

Of course, it is not always possible to turn the thing you love into paid work. A sensible compromise may be to participate in hobbies or voluntary work that allow you to do more of what you love and what the world needs.

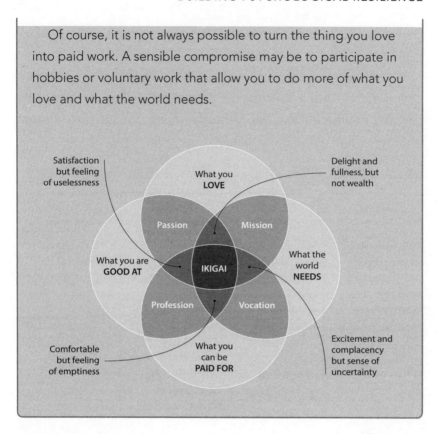

Realistic optimism

I have a real problem with the general notion of positive thinking. To my mind, what a lot of self-help and popular psychology call 'positive thinking'[*], in which someone is encouraged to ignore unpleasant feelings, looks a lot like denial and delusion. It contains too much of what I recognise as emotional suppression for it to be a sustainable approach to psychological health. In fact, avoiding dealing with difficult situations undermines resilience because you

---

* Not to be confused with Positive Psychology, which is an evidence-based psychological approach that focuses on enhancing individual strengths and capacities.

never benefit from the process of stress inoculation, skill development or mastery.

However, the concept of realistic optimism, in which you pay attention to negative outcomes but do not dwell on them, instead focusing on the growth opportunities, is associated with greater resilience than either a pessimistic or unrealistically optimistic viewpoint.

Scenario	Pessimist	Realistic optimist	Unrealistic optimist
You're walking home and it starts pouring with rain. Your feet are soaking wet. And you're hungry.	This is typical! It's been dry all day and it starts to rain NOW! Now I won't be able to wear these shoes tomorrow. Something bad always happens to me.	Well, this is sub-optimal. At least it didn't rain this afternoon when I was walking to the office. That would have been really bad. At least I will be home soon.	It's forecast to rain but I'm pretty sure it won't rain on me. Oh . . .

I often say that the attitude of the realistic optimist can be summed up in the phrase, 'At least it . . .' Here there is an acknowledgement of the undesired event that is balanced with the recognition that whatever is happening is manageable and/or that it will be over soon. This capacity to rationally reframe events is another example of cognitive flexibility.

Dealing with Failure

The fear of failure is a common anxiety I encounter in the therapy room. Perhaps it is the brilliant young medical student who develops panic attacks before her exams. Or the accountant who avoids leaving an organisation she hates afraid that others will think less of her. Or the couple that endures a loveless, sexless marriage because the stigma of divorce is too much to bear. A fear of failure can manifest in many forms, but ultimately it achieves a kind of paralysis that prevents the person from making important decisions in the direction of the things that they really want. If we can come to a place of tolerance with the idea of failing, we become much freer to take the kind of bold chances that we so admire in others.

Here's what we get wrong about failure and how to think about it differently:

- Failure as a noun: Often people will conceptualise a failed endeavour as an indication of a fixed aspect of their personality. Rather than saying, 'I did not succeed at this,' they say, 'I *am* a failure.' They use failure as a noun instead of a verb. It is important to understand that failure is an outcome of an attempt, not a feature of identity.
- 'I will always be a failure.': Similarly to seeing failure as a noun, there can be a sense in which a momentary failure will leave a lasting impression. This is an example of a cognitive bias known as fortune telling – behaving as though you can predict the future. Of course, this is impossible and you have no idea how things will turn out.
- 'No one else fails.': The problem here is that the stigma around failing means that few people are honest about the times when

they messed up or things didn't work out. This gives the impression that people in general are way more successful than they really are. Searching online for 'famous failures' is a good antidote for this. One of my favourites is J. K. Rowling's Harvard commencement speech.

- 'Everyone knows I have failed.': This is a feature of the 'spot-light effect' – the inaccurate belief that other people are paying close attention to what we are doing. In reality, most people are so concerned about themselves that they fail to notice what someone else is up to. Even when they do, they really won't care that much.

Making friends with failure

A recently published study provides more good news about failure – it is a pre-requisite of success. Dashon Wang and colleagues reviewed thousands of data sets on grant proposals and start-up investments and found that every winner begins as a loser; what is important is not avoiding failure but learning from it. Psychological resilience is the capacity to bounce back from difficulty. If you want to live a full life you must come to terms with the inevitability of failure and not allow it to steer you off course. Below are some approaches that have worked for me and my clients:

- Don't get too attached to the outcome. One of the most power-ful propensities of the human mind is the ability to become emotionally invested in future outcomes. This ability enables us to rehearse and visualise success, but also means that we feel genuine grief when plans are cancelled even when they are far off in the future. While we should *hope* for the best we should not *expect* everything to go according to plan. In most races there is only one winner – you need to be prepared for it not to be you.

- Prepare for failure. I don't mean *aim to fail*, but rather it is important for you to have considered what it might feel like to fail and what will happen if you do. Practitioners of classical stoicism see this kind or preparation for unwelcome outcomes as essential for maintaining emotional equilibrium in the face of defeat (i.e. resilience). Ask yourself the following questions:

1. What would failure look like in this situation?
2. How will it feel?
3. Is this the worst thing that has happened or could ever happen to me?
4. What can I do to reduce the risk of failing?
5. What will I have learned about myself or this activity even if I do fail?
6. How can I take this new knowledge forwards?

- Hone your self-compassion. Self-compassion can really be boiled down to showing yourself the same kind of consideration as you would someone else in a similar situation. For example, most people wouldn't turn to a friend who had failed a test and say, 'You are a total idiot and you should be ashamed of yourself' yet think nothing of saying the same to themselves, only compounding the emotional distress associated with the failure. Self-compassion offers a way out of this destructive cycle and is comprised of three elements:

1. Kindness: Treating yourself with the same care and decency as you would a friend.

2. A sense of common humanity: Understanding that every person on the planet has flaws, weaknesses and vulnerabilities. Everyone fails. Everyone messes up. You are no different.

3. Mindfulness: Acknowledging and accepting the reality of the present moment without wishing it were different.

Self-compassion is far from 'wishy-washy'; research shows that being able to show yourself compassion is linked to greater well-being, satisfaction, motivation, body-esteem and happiness. Rather than making you 'soft', self-compassion allows you to bounce back more quickly and more completely when things go wrong.

Takeaways
- Resilience is our psychological capacity to bounce back from challenging or traumatic situations. It is associated with lower stress-reactivity and reduced risk of depression.
- There is a genetic component to resilience, but the most important contribution is made by psychosocial factors that can be learned, developed and practised.
- Making time to invest in friendships and close relationships is probably the most important single thing you can do to improve your resilience. Be sure not to neglect the important people in your life. Make it a rule to schedule a regular catch-up, with penalties for cancelling, such as buying your friends an expensive dinner or agreeing to wash their car. If you know you are bad at keeping in touch, set yourself reminders. Put it in your diary to encourage yourself to make maintaining friendships at least as important as work.
- You become what you see or what you believe yourself to be, so surround yourself with people who live value-driven lives.

They don't need to have exactly the same values as you, but they should be people whom you think are good role models.

- Physical health contributes to psychological resilience (but you knew that already) so do what you can to eat well, exercise regularly, maintain good sleep and manage stress.
- Consider joining a local team or meet-up group. This can help to foster a sense of community and help you to meet new people. Whether it's hockey, walking or a book club, local interest groups are a great place to meet people and deepen connections.
- Avoid unnecessary risks but do not shy away from challenge. Keep challenging your brain with novelty and learning opportunities. Keep challenging your courage by practising vulnerability and honesty.
- Take some time to work out what you stand for. What do you want your life to mean? The meaning for your life does not have to be earth-shattering; personal and private definitions of meaning and success can be powerful. What positive difference could you make to your family, friends or your town?
- Try to cultivate an attitude of realistic optimism. This will help to prevent you from being blown over by small fluctuations in fortunes, saving your energy for when you need it most.

CHAPTER 13

Other Lifestyle Factors That Impact Brain Health

Building a healthy brain is all about reducing the risks and optimising the upsides of lifestyle factors on our brains and mental health. So far we have looked at some of the most well-known interventions, but there are some other, lesser-known activities that evidence suggests are important additions to a brain-healthy lifestyle.

Heat

The human body functions optimally at a core temperature of between 36.5 and 37.5°C. This temperature reflects the ideal conditions for the enzyme activity that underpins much of human metabolism, and is tightly controlled by various mechanisms of thermoregulation, including automatic responses such as vasodilation and constriction, shivering and sweating, as well as behaviours such as seeking out shade or putting on warmer clothes. This requirement for a precisely maintained core body temperature means that dramatic shifts in the ambient temperature that move the body out of this range, during a heatwave for example, create a significant physiological stress.

Yet practices that induce heat stress have been a part of traditional communities across the world for centuries, from the sweat lodges of indigenous Americans to the Turkish bath and the Russian banya. The Scandinavians are also well-known sauna bathing nations and now a flurry of research from Finland is beginning to show that saunas and heat stress have profound health benefits for the whole body and the brain.

How heat affects the brain

There are several ways in which heat exposure influences brain health. On page 237 you'll find practical ways to put this evidence into action in your own life.

Heat promotes neurogenesis Brain-derived neurotrophic factor (BDNF), the compound that stimulates the growth of new brain cells, is reliably increased through exercise (see page 146). Scientists also noticed that people who exercised in a warm environment had higher blood levels of BDNF than cool-room exercisers. Could the higher core body temperature induced from working out in a warm room account for these effects?

A team of Japanese researchers demonstrated this effect using an experimental design in which the participants acted as their own control group. This means that each person was first tested under one experimental condition before they were given time to return to their own biological baseline. They were then tested under the other condition. This procedure helps to eliminate any differences in the results that could be associated to natural variation between individual participants, and allows researchers to have more confidence that any significant change is due to the thing being tested. In this study the researchers looked at the difference in levels of BDNF when the participants were immersed up to the neck in hot water (42°C) or in water around body temperature (35°C) for 20 minutes. During the hot water condition the participants' core body temperature increased to 39.5 ± 0.6°C, which was associated with an increase in BDNF that was not seen in the lukewarm water condition. Additionally, levels of cortisol (a stress hormone) dropped significantly after hot water immersion. Incidentally, 42°C is roughly the temperature of a hot bath, suggesting that you may not need access to a sauna to reap the potential brain benefits of heat exposure.

Heat releases endorphins Opioids are a family of psychoactive substances that have potent analgesic (pain-relieving) effects. Prescription medications such as morphine, codeine and Fentanyl, as well as illegal drugs like cocaine and heroin, all act on the brain's opioid receptors. How is it that the brain has in-built receptors for these substances? Well, the brain produces its own endogenous opioids in the form of endorphins. As with the other opioids, endorphins suppress pain-signalling and produce feelings of euphoria. Endorphins are released in response to heat exposure.

Heat reduces inflammation C-reactive protein (CRP) is one of the most studied and robust markers of chronic systemic inflammation. A trial of over 2,000 healthy middle-aged men (aged 42–60 years) found an inverse relationship between the frequency of sauna use and blood levels of CRP, ie the more often these men used the sauna, the lower their markers of inflammation.

Heat reduces amyloid accumulation We have seen how neurodegenerative disorders such as dementia and cognitive impairment are associated with the accumulation of misfolded proteins such as amyloid beta. One of the ways that the body tries to limit and reduce this accumulation is through the glymphatic system (see page 71). Another way is simply through refolding the misfolded proteins. Heat shock proteins (HSPs) are a family of proteins produced when core body temperature rises. Many HSPs act as 'chaperones' to amyloid beta, helping to prevent misfolding or supporting refolding into its proper shape. If a protein is too damaged to be repaired, HSPs can also help to avoid accumulation by guiding the damaged protein into a pathway where it is broken down and recycled.

You can think of HSPs as the sensible friend on a night out, the one that calms everyone down (refolding), steps in to break up the fight (prevents accumulation) or just puts the troublemaker in a taxi and gets them out of there (recycling). In this way HSPs are neuro-protective and support the survival of brain cells even when a disease process has begun.

Heat as a potential treatment
So we know *how* heat can affect the brain, but is there any evidence of heat exposure as an effective treatment? Research is in its early stages but, so far, the results are promising.

Depression A small (28 participants) randomised controlled trial of unmedicated patients with mild depression investigated the effect of heat stress on the depressive symptoms. Half the group lay down for 15 minutes in a dry infrared sauna heated to 60°C, and then lay wrapped in a blanket for a further 30 minutes in a 28°C room. The control group spent the same 45 minutes lying in a 24°C room. Participants repeated this every day, Monday to Friday, for four weeks, totalling 20 sessions. At the end of the trial the participants who had received the thermal treatment had fewer physical symptoms, improved appetites and were more relaxed compared to the control group. Day-to-day these changes would be associated with improved quality of life for these individuals.

In a separate trial of 16 young people with a diagnosis of major depressive disorder (MDD), a single session of whole-body hyperthermia provided a significant antidepressant effect. Similarly, a double-blind randomised controlled trial of individuals with MDD in which they were warmed with infrared lamps until their core body temperature reached 38.5°C found that a single session of heat exposure produced a significant reduction in depression symptoms up to six weeks later.

Dementia and Alzheimer's disease The upregulation of BDNF and the chaperone action of HSPs suggest that heat stress may be protective against brain ageing, but what does the evidence show?

A prospective study is one in which a group of participants' health status is assessed at baseline and then tracked over several years. A Finnish trial used this type of design to investigate the impact of sauna use on men's dementia risk. What they found was truly incredible. Compared to men who used the sauna only once a week, men who sauna bathed four to seven times per week had a 66 per cent reduction in their risk of dementia and a 65 per cent risk reduction for Alzheimer's disease. This relationship remained even after the researchers adjusted for other factors such as smoking, alcohol consumptions, BMI and cholesterol.

The same research lab also found a similar effect for psychotic disorders, in which men who used the sauna four to seven times per week had a 77 per cent reduced risk of these illnesses.

> **Caution**
>
> Saunas are not for everyone: children, pregnant women, those with blood pressure disorders, heart disease/myocardial ischemia (including angina and unstable angina), people on certain medications and anyone who has difficulty regulating their body temperature are not advised to use saunas.

How Paying Attention Can Shape the Brain

I noted earlier that the more years you spend in education the lower your risk of developing dementia. There are several factors that might contribute to this phenomenon. We know that people who are able to undertake graduate and postgraduate study tend to come from wealthier families than those who do not, with the additional brain benefits that come from this good fortune. However, there is good evidence to suggest that the act of *paying attention* is one of the key components of this apparent protective effect of learning. In 2011 Dr Sara Lazar published a piece of research that changed our understanding of how thinking practices could influence not just the function, but also the physical structure of our brains.

In an earlier study in 2005 her team had compared the brains of meditators and otherwise healthy non-meditators. Meditation is the act of paying quiet and close attention to a word (such as a mantra), an action (like the breath) or an emotion (such as compassion). Brain scans showed that regular meditators had thicker brains (think 'cognitive reserve') compared to matched controls (people who were selected for their general similarity to the meditators, but who did not meditate). Notably, greater brain density was seen in the prefrontal cortex, which usually shrinks as we age. Lazar reported that the brains of the 40–50-year-old meditators were as healthy as the 20–30-year-old non-mediators. This observation raised a compelling question: Could meditation slow brain ageing?

Since this was a correlation it was not clear whether, for example, regular meditators did not also follow other lifestyle habits associated with better brain health. In order to be able to determine causality Lazar designed an experimental trial. In this follow-up trial 16 participants who were not regular meditators (i.e. they had not meditated in the last six months or had done fewer than four sessions in the last five years) had their brains scanned before commencing a 30-minute daily meditation programme for eight weeks. At the end of the study the participants' brains were scanned again and compared to their pre-trial assessments. Remarkably, even in this short time frame there were significant brain changes. Meditation practice:

- Stimulated growth in the left hippocampus (linked to better memory and emotion regulation).
- Increased density in the temporal-parietal junction (linked to processing our relationships with others).
- Reduced density in the amygdala, which in this trial correlated with reduced stress.

Why should meditation be able to change the brain? And how does this link to the health benefits – greater cognitive reserve – associated with more years of education? The answer lies in what happens in the brain when we *pay attention.*

Cells that fire together, wire together

When an event or a piece of information is especially important or relevant (meaningful) to us, or when we are in a state of greater autonomic arousal (readiness for action), the brain releases more of the neurotransmitters acetylcholine and dopamine at the synapses that were activated during that event. Acetylcholine* acts to strengthen the synapses, making them active and increasing the likelihood that they remain active over the long-term (a process called 'long-term potentiation'). The dopamine provides a sense of value, meaning or reward for the effort. That means that the next time we encounter a similar stimulus, those neurones are that little bit more ready to encode the information – they are ready to learn and grow. The more this cycle is repeated, the more active and connected the cells in that area become. So *paying attention* is actually one of the driving forces behind neuroplasticity (the capacity for your brain to reshape). Just the practice of concentrating on something can stimulate the release of compounds that can reshape your brain. How incredible is that? This is one of the reasons it is important to try to limit distractions if you want to boost your chances of learning new information.

Repetition strengthens neural networks, hardwiring that information into our brains. This can have positive and negative consequences. For example, when you are learning to ride a bike or drive a car the combination of the desire to succeed (motivation and meaning), the slight stress of being on the road (autonomic arousal) and the repetition of the movements, modulates the neurones associated with the actions of driving or keeping your balance on the

---

* Interestingly, there is some evidence that works against acetylcholine medication, such as amitriptyline, is associated with increased risk of dementia.

bike. Eventually, this encoding becomes built-in or 'hardwired' and the activity becomes automatic. On the negative side, this same process can undermine our psychological health. It means that the experience of repeated stress or trauma can lead to a reinforcing or hardwiring of those responses into the brain. Perhaps you get into the habit of self-criticism and do it so often that it becomes the automatic way that you think about yourself. Now you have a hard-wired circuit for self-criticism that can be difficult to change.*

While habits or familiar behaviours are wired into our brains – those pathways are already there and it takes very little effort to fire them up – when we encounter novel information our brains have to work hard to make sense of it and work out where it sits with the rest of everything else we already know. This additional brain effort is why old habits can be hard to break and why 'practice makes perfect'. But how can you use this information to your advantage?

1. Pay attention: Focus and attention increase the release of the neurotransmitters required for synaptic plasticity (aka neuro-genesis), priming the brain for learning.
2. Repetition: The more a thought or action is repeated the more the synapses are reinforced.
3. Novelty: The challenge of learning something new or being in a novel environment forces you to pay attention, driving a constant need for adaptation (neurogenesis).

People who have had many years of education have spent a lot of time *paying attention* to, and *repeating, novel* information, processes

---

* One of the core features of therapy is to help patients break unhelpful patterns, to diminish activation of these networks. More on the neuroscience of therapy in Chapter 17.

that contribute to cognitive reserve, the brain's pension plan. Whether it is ongoing learning, meditation or any other absorbing activity, honing your powers of attention might be an important component of the brain health toolkit.

Dental Health

We have looked at the impact of *what* you eat and *whether* you eat on your brain health, but there is one more food-related factor to consider. A familiar observation in dementia research is the poor dental condition of patients, who often have gum disease and/or missing teeth. It had been thought that, if there was a relationship between the two, it was that poor dentition made it difficult for people to eat nutritious foods, such as the crunchy vegetables that are associated with better brain health. This is a plausible assumption. However, recent developments in animal research and correlates in human brain tissue samples are leading researchers to follow new lines of investigation.

You may recall that there are a few exceptions to the extent of the blood–brain barrier (see page 29). A handful of areas in the brain called the 'circumventricular organs' actually have highly permeable membranes. This permeability allows them to play their important roles in maintaining homeostasis by monitoring the contents of the bloodstream and relaying this information to other areas of the brain. However, harmful compounds such as fragments of bacteria can access these areas and, when they do, they can trigger microglia, which then secrete pro-inflammatory cytokines, quinolinic acid and free radicals, all of which contribute to further inflammatory cascades.

Porphyromonas gingivalis (P.gingivalis) is the bacteria that causes gum disease (hence 'gingivitis'). It produces an enzyme (gingipains) that breaks down proteins (like gum tissue), increases the permeability of blood vessels and induces inflammation. In a series of elegant trials, an international research team examined the relationship between P.gingivalis and Alzheimer's disease. They found that:

- In animal trials, bacteria from diseased gums were able to travel to the brain. They did so in every case.
- The brains of mice with P.gingivalis infection accumulated more amyloid than non-infected mice. Further, mice with gum disease that was treated with a compound that inhibits gingipains had less amyloid in their brains than untreated mice.
- The areas of inflammation in the infected mouse brains were the same as those in human Alzheimer's brain tissue samples.
- Gingipains were present in nearly all (96 per cent) of the brains of human Alzheimer's patients and the level of gingipains in these brains correlated to Alzheimer's severity.

Importantly, recent data has highlighted a more nuanced picture of the activity of amyloid beta. Though the clumps of this protein are a characteristic of Alzheimer's disease progression, drugs that clear amyloid from the brain do not result in improvement. Further, animal trials have pointed to a *protective* effect of amyloid beta against bacterial infection, including P.gingivalis. It may be, then, that amyloid beta initially arrives to help *fight off* bacterial infection in the brain. However, if the infection is prolonged (such as chronic gum disease), eventually the amyloid ends up clogging up the system and doing more harm than good. Imagine a fire starts in a small bakery on a narrow street. One fire engine arrives and starts to put out the flames. But then another arrives, and another. Soon the road is so blocked with fire engines it becomes impossible to reach the fire. The flames blaze through the bakery and start to burn the neighbouring buildings, and the same pattern of too many fire engines blocking the roads continues. This may be analogous to the process of damage in Alzheimer's disease, where the amyloid (fire crew) initially arrives to fight off the bacteria (fire) but causes unintended harm. Maybe all this time researchers have been looking at the damage in the brain and blaming the firefighters without recognising the original source of the fire (bacteria or other chronic infection).

So now we have a new model to describe the relationship between gum disease and Alzheimer's disease that looks something like this:

Development of gum disease through a combination of poor diet and poor dental hygiene.

Transfer of P.gingivalis and/or gingipains to the brain e.g. via the trigeminal or olfactory nerve, circumventricular organs or impaired BBB (from systemic inflammation).

Stimulation of microglia – production of pro-inflammatory cytokines, quinolinic acid, free radicals.

Brain cells are damaged by the gingipains *and* the inflammatory products, leading to further inflammation and cell death.

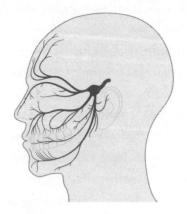
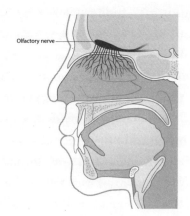

Olfactory nerve

It may be that recurrent exposure to many infectious agents triggers the inflammatory response seen in Alzheimer's disease. For example, even urinary tract infections, bacterial infections that affect the urethra, bladder and kidneys, are a risk factor for later developing dementia. Importantly, gum disease is a common infection that, unlike many others, can be easily prevented and treated.

What to do
- Be sure to register with your local dentist.
- Brush your teeth twice a day with a fluoride toothpaste, for at least two minutes.
- Don't rinse your mouth with water after brushing. Instead, spit out any excess toothpaste. This allows any residual fluoride to continue working.
- Floss at least once per day (your dental hygienist can show you the most effective way to do this).
- Be sure to visit your dentist regularly, they can monitor for signs of gum disease and advise on treatment.
- Parents must encourage good brushing routines in children. Under-sevens should be supervised to ensure they are brushing

properly. Children should attend annual dentist appointments from the age of 18 months.

- Reduce consumption of foods containing free (added) sugars, such as chocolate, sweets, cakes, sweetened cereals, sauces and sugar-sweetened beverages (see Chapter 7).
- Make an appointment to see your dentist if your notice blood when you brush your teeth, have tooth sensitivity, develop dark spots on your teeth or notice an unpleasant taste in your mouth.
- Stop smoking, or try to cut back.
- Keep alcohol consumption to within healthy limits (see page 122).

Takeaways

- Heat stress upregulates BDNF production, thereby supporting neurogenesis.
- Heat reduces markers of inflammation in a dose-response manner.
- Regular sauna use is associated with reduced depression incidence and reduced risk of dementia and Alzheimer's disease, in a dose-response manner.
- In trials, 20 minutes of 80°C heat is an effective dose. If you are new to sauna use, build up your heat tolerance slowly, starting with just a few minutes per session. Try to go once or twice a week.
- If you do not have access to a sauna, the temperature-raising effect of 30 minutes in a hot bath and/or exercise may also confer at least some of these benefits.
- Sauna use is not without risk. If you are part of a vulnerable group, please seek medical advice as to whether it is safe for you to use saunas.
- Attention is one of the driving forces behind neuroplasticity. If you want to increase your chances of successful learning try to limit any distractions and give the task or activity your full attention.

- Meaning motivates attention. We are better learners of information that feels more personally relevant to us. When undertaking learning a new skill try to remind yourself of *why* it is important to you.
- Repetition strengthens neural networks. The more you repeat something the more it will be hardwired into your brain. Meditation and mindfulness practices strengthen our attention 'muscles' and can reshape the brain in healthy ways. Try the 4-4-8 breath practice on page 169 if you are new to these sorts of attention practices.
- Stay curious – novel experiences and learning something new help to stimulate new connections in the brain, building cognitive reserve, but it's not just formal education that can provide these benefits. There are thousands of hours of free classes and courses available online, or try learning a new skill in your local area. A list of online learning resources is provided on page 317.
- Gum disease may be a significant factor in the progress of Alzheimer's disease, which means looking after your teeth offers an accessible way of reducing your risk.

CHAPTER 14

How Social Media and
Technology Affect the Brain

We have adopted the use of smartphones faster than any technology in the history of our species. Aside from concerns about blue light exposure, the near-ubiquity of screen-based devices (laptops, notebooks, smartphones, smart watches, etc.) and the correlational rise in psychological distress, especially among young people, has led to concerns and claims that the two might be linked. Could devices be driving the apparent rise in mental illness?

Initially, there were worries that simply the act of being on a device was harmful. However, recent research is pointing to the *nature* of use, in combination with individual personality factors, as being the determining factor as to whether users will be better or worse off.

Social Networking Sites

Social networking sites like Facebook, Twitter and Instagram are designed to capture as much of our attention as possible, and that's not just my opinion. Famously, the former president of Facebook, Sean Parker, said of building these applications:

To really understand it, that thought process was all about 'how do we consume as much of your time and conscious attention as possible?' And that means that we need to give you a little dopamine hit ... it's a social validation feedback loop ... you're exploiting a vulnerability in human psychology.

One of those vulnerabilities is our innate tendency to compare ourselves to others, and never before have we had as much access to material with which to do this. Sites such as Instagram contain billions of images, many of them depicting an idealised body type or lifestyle. Since people rarely use social media to post negative or mundane content, this unrelenting showreel of perfection can contribute to a distorted view that 'everyone is doing better than me'. It also increases the likelihood of making upwards social comparisons (see below), which can undermine self-esteem.

Watch out for negative comparisons!
Humans have an innate need to know where we fit in the social hierarchy and to attempt to elevate our status. We do this, in part, by comparing an aspect of ourselves, whether a physical trait, psychological quality, talent, ability or wealth, to others. Social comparison theory describes the pattern of these comparisons and the impact they have on well-being. Broadly, the comparisons are split into two: downwards and upwards.

In a downwards comparison, you choose an ability, say public speaking, and compare yourself to others whom are not as good as you. This downward comparison (literally 'looking down' on others) can have the effect of temporarily making you feel better about yourself. However, it is an incredibly fragile basis for self-esteem. It also underlies some of the uglier elements of social life – the way that commenters pile in on public mistakes; implicit in delighting in others' misfortune is the wish to elevate our own self-concept.

An upwards comparison is the opposite process. Here you find someone whom you consider to be superior to you on this quality, such as a professional motivational speaker. In this case, the upwards comparison can follow one of two routes:

1. Motivation: 'One day I could be as good as that.'
2. Demoralisation: 'I'll never be as good as that. What's the point?'

Importantly, the more valuable or idealised the skill, quality or person is, the more compelled you will be to engage in upwards comparisons, and the greater pressure to try to achieve 'improvement' (whether that is realistic or not).

Social comparison is an ongoing automatic process whether we are online or meeting people in real life, though evidence indicates that people engage in more upwards comparisons online than they do in the real world. Engaging in too many upwards comparisons increases the risk of feeling demoralised because the repeated experience of feeling 'less than' under-mines self-esteem. Be mindful about whom you choose to compare yourself to and, online, how many accounts you follow that make you feel worse about yourself or your circumstances.

In a paper published in 2019 researchers conducted three studies to test a series of hypotheses about the relationship between the use of social networking sites (such as Facebook), self-esteem and depression, crucial components of psychological well-being. In the first experiment participants were split into three groups:

1. Presented with online information about people via Facebook.
2. Presented with online information about staff members of a university.
3. Not presented with any information.

Participants in groups one and two were then asked to write down everything they could remember about the first five people they were presented with. Later all three groups completed questionnaires designed to assess self-esteem. Those in groups one and two expressed lower performance-related self-esteem than those in group three – the control condition.

Next the research team conducted two questionnaire studies. The first asked participants about their Facebook activity, and assessments of social comparison tendencies, self-esteem and depressive symptoms. They then processed the data using statistical analysis procedures that can identify the influence of one factor on another. They reported that passive Facebook use – just watching/scrolling without actively posting – was associated with greater social comparison, lower self-esteem and greater depression.

The final trial in the series was an online survey in which participants, all users of a business networking site similar to LinkedIn, also completed the questionnaires from the previous study. A mediation analysis showed the following pattern:

Passive Facebook use → greater social comparison on ability → lower self-esteem → greater depression

This was just one trial but it replicates and extends previous findings. Exposure to information about other people's lives triggers social comparison in a predominately upwards (negative) direction.

Furthermore, passive use (of Facebook in this case) increases opportunities for social comparison, driving upwards comparisons, resulting in poorer self-evaluations and worsened mood.

What about the flipside? Can social networking sites be a force for psychological good? A new study of school girls in the UK suggests they can. In this study researchers gave girls aged 14–17 a list of positive female role models to follow in their own stated areas of interest.* Later in the school year the girls were interviewed about their aspirations, mental health and how their use of social media had changed over the study period. They found that:

- At the end of the study girls were more likely to see social media as a platform for education and learning as well as entertainment.
- Following a more diverse range of positive female role models disrupted what they were presented with each day in the 'explore' sections of their feeds. They were presented with a greater diversity of content that related to their interests and passion, which provided opportunities for positive action, like applying for scholarships.
- Participation in the study highlighted the impact of social media on mental health for some participants, encouraging them to be more proactive with online self-care, such as taking breaks from social media and unfollowing accounts that undermined their self-esteem.
- It helped the girls to visualise their own future career possibilities and expanded their world views, helping to break out of the all-too-common 'echo chamber' of social media.

* I was deeply honoured to find that I am featured on the list:
https://www.thefemalelead.com/transform-your-feed

In summary, social media can have positive or negative effects depending on the nature of use. Below are some tips to help you make the most positive use of your time online.

Positive use

- Be active. Engage positively and compassionately with friends' pictures and stories. Use social media as an additional element to your existing relationships. Show appreciation for content and information that you find valuable. Try to be purposeful with your engagement – go online for a reason (like posting an update) rather than just to fill time while you're waiting in a queue.

- Less intense. Treat social media like a condiment rather than a main meal. Avoid spending several hours a day passively scrolling. You may find it useful to download an app that tracks your usage time, so that you know how much time you spend on social media. Set yourself a reasonable daily limit and try to stick to it!

- Different opinions. It is easy to get stuck in an echo chamber online, only engaging with people who agree with your point of view and avoiding opinions that differ from yours. However, engaging respectfully with people who disagree with you can help broaden your knowledge and your appreciation for others' perspectives. It will also show you how the same information can be spun for different audiences. Try following smart people who have opinions that differ from your own.

- Support. Social media can often look like a 'showreel' of people living perfect lives, but being honest and letting people know when you need help is an important part of healthy relationships. Connecting with your friends when you are struggling with a situation can give you access to valuable support.

- Avoid body comparisons. The evidence is very strong that viewing hundreds of images of other people's bodies makes us feel worse about ourselves. It may be good for you to unfollow accounts where this is the majority of content, even if you like the account holder. It's not about disliking them but prioritising your well-being.

Impaired Processing

It makes intuitive sense that we may be affected, positive or negatively, by technology with which we have direct contact, but a fascinating study showed that simply looking at your phone may have negative effects on brain power.

In an elegantly designed study 548 participants were asked to sit down at a computer to complete a cognitively demanding task. There were three experimental conditions, but the only thing that differed was what the participants were asked to do with their phones:

- Place it on the desk, face down.
- Put it in a pocket or bag, within the room.
- Leave it in another room, out of reach and sight.

When they analysed performance on the task, working memory and fluid intelligence was worst in the 'desk' condition, better in the 'pocket/bag' condition and best when phones were completely out of reach. Strikingly, most participants, across all the conditions, reported that they did not think that the location of their phone impacted their performance. They were unaware of the difference it was making.

These results are a function of cognitive capacity – the principle that your brain has a finite amount of available processing power at any moment. The outcome suggests that when your phone is nearby or noticeable, a portion of your processing power (attention) is devoted to it, perhaps trying to resist the temptation to pick it up, or wondering what might be happening online. This reduces the available processing power for other activities. The message here is simple: if you want to give your full attention to something or someone, put your phone away.

Typing

I am one of the few people I know who still uses a pen and paper diary for organising my day. I've tried using the integrated calendar on my smartphone, but the events don't seem to 'stick' in my head in the way that they do when I write them down. Some recent studies seem to back up my observation and the effect relates to depth of processing.

Psychologists Pam Mueller and Daniel Oppenheimer were interested in whether there was any difference in test performance depending on the method of note-taking. In the trial 65 students viewed five TED Talks and were asked to take notes on them either by hand or by typing on a laptop. They then spent around 30 minutes engaging in distractor tasks, designed to take their attention away from the talks they had just been watching, before being tested on the material. The first observation was that the style of notes differed. They found that students taking laptop notes were more likely to record the information word-for-word. In comparison, students who took longhand notes were forced to put the information into their own words and thereby engaged in a deeper level of cognitive processing. The test results showed significantly better conceptual application (how the concepts behaved in the real world) and better recall for the longhand note-takers. What was even more striking was that, even when the students were allowed to *reread* their notes, the longhanders still outperformed the typists.

Research with children shows that handwriting engages more areas of the brain than typing and may support language development. And students who wrote about their learning (compared to students who were just quizzed on it) significantly improved their critical thinking skills.

While the biological mechanisms are still being worked out, there certainly seems to be something about the process of writing by hand that recruits more areas of the brain and improves performance on a range of areas. This might be most useful for students or when you are trying to remember important information, perhaps for a best man's speech or a presentation at work. Some element of pen-and-paper note-taking may help to enhance your memory performance.

Broken connections

Researchers Kostadin Kushlev and colleagues invited 304 participants to take part in a cafe-based study in which people were invited to have lunch with friends or family. Believing they were taking part in a study about dining experiences, all participants agreed to complete a one-question survey afterwards. However, half the group were told that the survey would be texted to them and therefore they would need to keep their phones on the tables with notifications turned on. The other half were told that the survey would be paper-based, and were asked to turn their phones to silent and leave them in a basket under the table. When they were later asked about their experience at the meal, those with their phones on the table reported less enjoyment compared to the other group.

The Health Risks of Fake News and How Critical Thinking Can Help

Fake news is bad for your health. That is not hyperbole: a study from Manchester Metropolitan University found that people who had low 'information discernment' (they did not check the reliability of the information they received) had a flawed response to threat, which elevated stress levels and harmed physical and mental health.

We are innately drawn to the emotional significance of an incoming message *over* the facts and evidence. The effect is so powerful that some trials have shown that presenting people with real evidence that contradicts their strongly held beliefs can result in them simply doubling down on those beliefs. This has serious consequences when false beliefs influence important decisions.

The story of Belle Gibson is a pertinent example. A critical appraisal of her claims would perhaps have led more people to question whether there were any proven cases of people treating cancer with a vegan diet. But Belle presented a very emotionally compelling story, had a large online following and seemed like a nice person.

As well as the risk to individuals, insufficient critical thinking creates serious problems at a population level. For example, though several high-quality reviews have now debunked the claim that the measles vaccine causes autism in children, rates of vaccination continue to fall, leading to outbreaks of the highly contagious and dangerous disease in areas where it had once been eradicated.

Level up your thinking

Primary and secondary school education is dominated by rote learning. Consequently, school children show low information discernment. To counteract this, one of the first modules university students often study is 'Critical Thinking Skills'. This is intended to shift them out of a mode of passive learning into being active, inquisitive thinkers. Critical thinking skills encourage you to interrogate the validity and veracity of the information you are consuming, and to question your assumptions. With the now unfettered access to infinite streams of information, statistics, opinions and claims granted to us by the Internet, critical thinking skills have never been more important.

Below is a list of questions you can use as a framework for your own critical thinking skills and to help protect you from falling for fake news and misinformation:

Who said it?	Your relationship to or opinion of the person making the claim will influence your response to it. How positive you feel about someone, or the more similar they are to you, the more you are likely to believe them. Remember that sometimes nice, likeable people are wrong, or lying.
What did they say?	What is the claim? How does it sit with your observations? How does it fit with previous information or knowledge in this area?
Is what they are saying a fact or an opinion?	Sometimes opinions are presented as facts. Of course, people can and should share hypotheses but it should be clear whether what they are saying is demonstrable fact, informed guess or opinion.
Are they a legitimate authority?	Is the person in a position that would grant them access to the information needed to make the claim?

What else would need to be true for this statement to be correct?	'Steel man' the claim. Steel-manning an argument is a way of testing the strength of the case. For example, if someone says 'gluten is harmful for everyone,' what else would need to be true for this case to stand? Everyone who ate gluten would need to be in poor health, and countries that consume high levels of gluten-containing foods would have to have high recorded rates of illness. If this is not the case, then it cannot be that gluten is bad for *everyone*.
Why did they say it?	What is the other person's investment in the outcome? What do they stand to gain? Is there a conflict of interests? Gaining from a position does not automatically invalidate it, but it should make us more cautious about accepting it.
When did they say it?	Might they be trying to influence an outcome or public opinion?
Can they back it up?	If they are making a factual claim, what evidence do they use to support it? Does the evidence appear sound?
Is there a moral imperative?	Most people who are sure of the factual validity of what they are saying do not have to appeal to emotions. If someone invokes a moral imperative ('smart people agree with me') that may be a clue that the foundations of their argument are not so strong.

Have better debates

The increased and speedy access to opinions has also increased our opportunities to argue. This in itself is no bad thing; reasoned debate is an important means of strengthening ideas and promoting action. However, without a thoughtful approach it is easy for debates and disagreements to descend into insults and name-calling, which promotes perceived stress, hostility and retaliatory escalation.

In 2008 the computer scientist Paul Graham wrote a prescient essay, 'How to Disagree', in which he outlined a framework for how to debate effectively and respectfully. Expressed as a pyramid (see below) the lower levels represent the weaker forms of argument. The arguments improve in quality as you move up the pyramid.

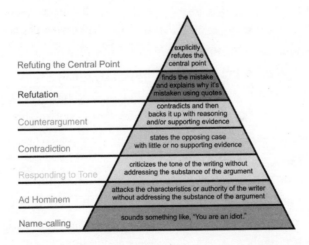

At the bottom is name-calling, attacks on the person and tone aimed at undermining their character or embarrassing them. This amounts to little more than bullying. Contradiction and counter-arguments begin to challenge the original position but it is refutation and refutation of the central point, with strong evidence, that will move the discussion forward towards a resolution.

Argue in good faith Entering a discussion in good faith means presenting your case while being willing to be proved wrong and, consequently, to change your position or amend your thinking. It means remaining open-minded to the possibility that you might be wrong. If you are unwilling to do this, it is probable that what you are seeking is dominance and capitulation rather than a true debate, an attitude that can lead you to behave in disrespectful ways that undermine your position and the case you are trying to make.

Most of the issues facing humanity are complex and do not have simple solutions that will make everyone happy. Reasoned debate is our only hope of reaching a workable resolution. Disagreeing with someone's ideas should not mean dismissing them as a person. You can disagree with someone's ideas or beliefs and still respect them as a human being. You should expect the same in return. Finally, expect to compromise. Trying to hold fast to an extreme position will only result in stalemate or long-term instability.

Takeaways

- There is as yet no consensus on whether smartphone technology is good for us or not. It is likely that the *way* that we interact with and use technology is the deciding factor on its impact on mental health.
- Remembering that social comparison happens every time we are confronted with information about other people's lives may help to buffer us from its effects.
- People tend to make more upwards comparisons on social media than they do in real life, which may be linked to the 'showreel' nature of most people's social media content.

- The risk of upwards comparisons does seem to increase with the amount of time spent on social media. Though the direction of causality is unclear (does sadness drive greater use or does greater use drive sadness?), it would seem wise to try to exert some control over the amount of time spent on social networking sites. Consider setting a curfew or downloading an app that limits your access to these sites.
- Try not to get into the habit of simply scrolling through social media as this kind of passive use is associated with poorer mental health outcomes.
- Following a diverse range of positive role models may have beneficial effects on mental health, especially for young people.
- If you are trying to focus on some deep work (such as revision or analysing data) it may help to put your smartphone out of sight and out of easy reach. Leave it in another room or in a lockable drawer.
- Phones may interfere with real-world social opportunities. Agree with friends to keep phones out of sight when you catch up. Leave them in a bag or pocket, not out on the restaurant table.
- Try to have a least one 'phone-free' journey per week. Decide not to use your phone on the way home from work, for example. You could read a book or simply observe what is happening around you instead.
- If you're revising or preparing for an important presentation consider writing out your notes by hand to help improve retention. Additionally, a handwritten journal can help you work through complex ideas and difficult emotions.
- Falling for fake news is bad for our psychological well-being. Critical thinking can help protect us from falling foul of misinformation.

- Critical thinking means interrogating the argument being put forward and, importantly, challenging your own assumptions. Use the questions on page 249 as a framework for improving your critical thinking.
- When engaging in a debate, take care to engage with the central point and avoid lower levels of argument.

CHAPTER 15

Money Matters

Money and mental health are intimately linked, and the relationship is bidirectional: concerns about money can contribute to stress, eroding mental health, and, conversely, being emotionally unwell may limit the ability to work, manage money, access to treatment and services, or make you more prone to risky spending. The difficulties around money are made even more complicated by the social norms around talking about it. Discussing money, at least in the UK, is seen as rude or inappropriate. Consequently, seeking help or advice about money management can feel deeply shameful. Even in clinic, when people have already told me intimate details about a secret drug habit or the eating disorder they can still struggle to discuss a personal debt or troubling spending habit, so intense is the social moratorium around money.

Money is a key marker of social status, and humans are acutely sensitive to where we fit in the social hierarchy (as seen in our tendency for social comparison). Being perceived as 'lower' on the social ladder is associated with feelings of shame, inadequacy and poorer self-esteem.

Money is, of course, the means by which we get our most fundamental needs – food, clothing, a safe place to live – met. Thus the risk of being without or losing money is an existential threat; it makes us feel incredibly vulnerable. Again, a sense of vulnerability or neediness is closely associated with feelings of shame; it makes us feel small and helpless and we are strongly motivated to avoid such emotional experiences, reinforcing the aversion to discussing money. However, the impact of money problems on psychological health and stress means that it is essential that we find a way to reduce the stigma around these conversations and make it easier to ask for and access help.

Many parents teach their children how to check they have been given the correct change, but few teach their children how to budget, save and avoid debt (indeed this is often something that they struggle with themselves). Neither is financial management taught at school. In effect this leaves us all at the mercy of commercial entities, which are, of course, invested in encouraging us to *spend* money, for guidance on what to do with the money we receive. Frighteningly, marketers are well-versed in the powerful psychological tricks that are effective at parting us from our cash. In a bid to redress this imbalance of power, I have outlined some of these tactics on the following pages, along with some information about how to improve your relationship with money. Unfortunately, it's not possible to give you a full financial overhaul in just a few pages, but hopefully raising your awareness of the impact of money on mental health will help you to take action in a positive direction.

How Companies Part You from Your Money

Psychologists cannot read minds (I promise) but the scientific study of Psychology and Behavioural Economics does provide powerful insights into our unconscious biases and irrational decision-making, and the often imperceptible tricks or 'nudges' that can shape a person's behaviour without them knowing. By utilising this knowledge, large organisations really can 'read your mind' and make you more likely to behave in specific ways.*

Changes in tobacco packaging and advertising are an impressive example of how influential these behavioural nudges can be. Smoking is a leading cause of preventable death, illness, disability and hospital admissions, and governments, public health organisations and charities are invested in reducing smoking rates. Rather than facing an outright ban, smokers have found themselves subject to a range of much more subtle techniques designed to discourage the habit:

• large health warnings on packets
• plain, unbranded packaging
• bans on smoking advertising

These measures do not limit an individual's access or freedom to purchase cigarettes, but they are successful in reducing the attractiveness of smoking and making smokers more cognizant of the health risks, thereby making them less *likely* to make the purchase. A Cochrane Review – recognised as the international gold standard for public health research – concluded that standardised (unbranded) packaging effectively reduced the appeal of cigarettes. Unbranded cigarettes were also judged as tasting worse and being of poorer quality than when

---

* Governments and corporate organisations face a moral and ethical dilemma when utilising behavioural nudges in the public sphere. Is it right to influence someone's behaviour, without their knowledge and consent, even if it is for their own good? Is it acceptable to use nudges for personal profit?

they were in the branded pack. This demonstrates the power of branding on our perception and enjoyment of a product.

So behavioural nudges really work. Here are some other money-related behavioural nudges you may encounter:

Online

- Check out the logos of the retailer Amazon, travel company TUI and catalogue store Argos. Notice anything? This is an example of 'priming' – the curved upwards line is reminiscent of a smile. This subtle allusion has been shown to increase positive feeling towards a brand and increase your likelihood of purchasing from them.

On the high street

- The 99: since readers of the Latin alphabet (e.g. English speakers) read from left to right, your brain will 'anchor' at the first number. So an item that costs £9.99 *feels* much cheaper than one priced at £10.
- The scarcity principle: 'Last Chance', 'Sale Ending Soon', 'Limited Edition', 'Don't Miss Out!' . . . marketers utilise the idea of scarcity to encourage sales because a) something that is scarce feels more valuable and b) it motivates our Fear of Missing Out (FOMO).

In the supermarket

- Eye level is buy level: Your eye is naturally drawn to products at eye level. Items placed here are the ones on which supermarkets make the highest margin i.e. the ones they want you to buy. Look down – the cheaper products are positioned on the lower shelves.

- Gold or silver gilding on labels both catches the eye and conveys a sense of luxury about the product. You are more likely to notice it and will be more willing to pay a higher price.
- End-of-aisle displays: Manufacturers pay a premium to supermarkets to promote products at the end of the aisle. Not only are these areas of the supermarket the ones with the highest footfall, but evidence shows that 'end cap' displays significantly increase sales.
- The decoy effect: See the box below for this beautiful example of irrationality in action.

The decoy effect

In marketing a 'decoy' is an item priced in such a way as to make the higher-priced item appear more desirable and good value for money. Let's imagine you go into a store to buy a bottle of water.

Small	Large
500 ml	1 litre
£1	£3

In this scenario, most people would choose the lower-priced option. However, imagine when entering the store you were presented with the following options:

Small	Medium	Large
500 ml	750 ml	1 litre
£1	£2.60	£3

> In comparison to the 750ml bottle, the large bottle of water feels like a bargain. You get an extra 250ml of water for 'only' 40p. Research tells us that the decoy effect is incredibly effective at nudging shoppers to pay for the higher-priced item. We fall for it all the time.

At home

- The 30-, 60- or 90-day free trial isn't just the retailer being generous; they are tapping into the 'endowment effect' – the way in which we are more willing to pay for, or less willing to part with, something that we already possess.
- Intangible products: the 'law of reciprocity' means that if someone gives us something, we feel a social pressure to give them something in return, which is why insurance companies are happy to bear the cost of that 'free' pen or soft toy; it increases the likelihood that you will feel compelled to buy their products.

Gambling

Gambling is a popular activity in the UK. According to a 2019 survey by the Gambling Commission, half of all men and 41 per cent of women had gambled in the previous four weeks. Gambling can be an incredibly compulsive activity because it takes advantage of a number of psychological vulnerabilities and cognitive biases such as:

1. Reward: Simply the opportunity to win increases dopamine activity in the brain, prompting continuation of the behaviour.

However, gambling utilises a very specific type of feedback called 'variable reward'. Psychological research dating back to the 1950s demonstrates that humans respond most compulsively to rewards that are intermittent or unpredictable (sometimes I win, sometimes I lose).

2. The gambler's fallacy is a feature of the fact that humans are innately bad at understanding probabilities. For example, I flip a coin 10 times. The probability of the first flip landing heads up is ½ or 50/50. If I flip nine heads in a row, the probability of the tenth flip landing heads up is still 50/50, but the gambler's fallacy means that, after having a streak of heads ups, I will *believe* that a tails outcome will be more likely.

3. Optimism bias: The idea that 'I will be the lucky one'.

The combination of these, and other, compelling processes means that gambling addiction, and the debt that can accompany it, poses a significant risk to mental health. It is estimated that just under 1 per cent of over 16s in the UK suffer with problem gambling. There are no quick solutions to addressing a gambling addiction, but it is important to try to address the issue as soon as possible. The screening questions in the box below will give you an indication of whether you might be at risk. If you think you might have a gambling problem, please refer to the support resources on page 318.

- Do you bet more than you can afford to lose?
- Do you need to gamble with larger amounts of money to get the same feeling?

- Have you tried to win back money you have lost ('chasing losses')?
- Have you borrowed money or sold anything to get money to gamble?
- Have you wondered whether you have a problem with gambling?
- Has your gambling caused you any health problems, including feelings of stress or anxiety?
- Have other people criticised your betting or told you that you have a gambling problem (regardless of whether or not you thought it was true)?
- Has your gambling caused any financial problems for you or your household?

- Have you ever felt guilty about the way you gamble or what happens when you gamble?

Score 0 for each time you answer 'never'.
Score 1 for each time you answer 'sometimes'.
Score 2 for each time you answer 'most of the time'.
Score 3 for each time you answer 'almost always'.
If your total score is 8 or higher, you may be a problem gambler.

SOURCE NHS: www.nhs.uk/live-well/healthy-body/gambling-addiction

Takeaways

- Money worries are a significant contributor to the burden of chronic stress and the relationship between money and psychological difficulties is bidirectional: money worries can promote or worsen mental health concerns, and mental illness can make it difficult to manage money responsibly.

- Marketers employ numerous sophisticated strategies to capitalise on our cognitive biases and heuristics. Being aware of them *may* help you to avoid spending more money than you intended.
- Use a list when you go shopping and stick to it.
- Try to avoid purchasing non-essential items on credit. The stress of paying off the debt will likely outlive the pleasure of the purchase.
- Gambling is a common activity that most people enjoy without coming to any harm. However, for some people, problem gambling and the debt that can come with it bring significant psychological risks. If you think you might have a gambling problem, please speak to someone and seek professional support. Resources are provided on page 318.
- Most local authorities offer services to help people manage their money, including advice on budgeting and managing debt. Contact your local council or go to www.moneyadviceservice.co.uk for details of local and international debt advice services, budget planners and savings calculators.

CHAPTER 16

Better Problem-Solving

Simply feeling that you have control over a situation can reduce the amount of stress you experience and managing stress is a crucial component of protecting your long-term brain health.

For some years I ran a therapy service in what was then Europe's largest women's prison. It would be neither inaccurate nor unfair to describe the prison system as the largest provider of psychiatric care in the UK. Though the prevalence of personality disorder in the general population is estimated to be between 5 and 10 per cent, it may exceed 50 per cent in prisoners. As a service manager, I trained in Dialectical Behaviour Therapy (DBT) to help address the mental health needs of my clients. DBT is a specialist treatment developed by psychologist Marsha Linehan to help people with a diagnosis of borderline personality disorder with the poor distress tolerance, emotion regulation and interpersonal skills that are often a feature of this diagnosis. It achieves this by combining cognitive behavioural therapy with mindfulness to help patients reduce emotional reactivity and gain some objectivity over their thoughts.

Though it was designed with a specific population in mind, I have found DBT's problem-solving skills to be a useful framework for patients without this diagnosis. Working through the steps can be useful in adding clarity to situations that can feel overwhelming and confusing. I offer them here in the hope that they may help you to work through difficult situations as and when they arise.

First it is important to be clear about what type of problem you are attempting to solve. Here is a list of common problems:

Type	Example
One-off problems	You realise that you have double-booked your plans for tomorrow night. It's impossible to do both so you need to cancel one.
People or situations that are habitually bad for you	You have a friend who is a 'bad influence'. You want to cut back on your drinking but they say you are boring if you don't drink. You always end up drinking too much when you go out with them.
People or situations that you find painful so you avoid them	You have a difficult relationship with a sibling so you avoid family events so that you don't have to see them.
Recurring problems	You agreed to take the minutes for the weekly team meeting. A few months in, your workload has increased and you no longer have the time to write up the minutes.
Long-term problems	You and your partner keep bickering. It's been going on for a while and is starting to make you really unhappy.

Repeated failures to stop harmful or ineffective behaviours	You regularly have deadlines to meet but can't seem to get a handle on your chronic procrastination.

All of these problems are solvable. The solutions may look different, and some of the solutions will require the courage to have some difficult conversations (see page 196), but they can be solved. Here are the four ways to tackle any problem:

1. Solve the problem (in a way that respects yourself and anyone else involved*).
2. Change your perception or attitude to the problem.
3. Learn to tolerate the problem: radical acceptance.
4. Stay miserable.

Solve the Problem

This sounds obvious, but this first step is really an invitation to you to commit to the task of resolving the problem. Often when there is a troubling issue in our lives we can be fully aware of it without committing to do anything about it. We may even construct plausible sounding 'reasons' why we can't address the issue:

> 'There's no point in talking to them. They would never listen.'

---

* Consistently demonstrating self-respect is one of the foundations of basic self-esteem, contributing to the inner sense that, fundamentally, you are a decent person. It may be more convenient to avoid or evade certain difficult situations, but the damage that this kind of behaviour can do to your well-being means it is really not worth it.

'I've never done that before.'

'They might be upset if I tell them.'

'It's scary.'

All of these statements may be true, but that does not make them a valid reason not to at least attempt to solve the problem. One of the factors that interferes with the idea of solving a problem, especially a difficult one, is the 'status quo bias'. Perhaps this has been a problem that has existed in your family for generations. Perhaps no one has ever dealt with it. If everyone else has managed to avoid having to deal with it, why should you be the one that has to? Because now it is your problem and by choosing not to address it, you are actively choosing to hold on to the problem for a while longer. Why would you choose that for yourself?

One way to help build the resolve required to address the problem is to identify the pain that it creates in your life. If we take the 'bad influence' friend as an example, identifying the pain might look like this:

- I am worried about the amount that I drink and I want to make positive changes to protect my future physical and mental health.
- It upsets me that this person doesn't support me wanting to look after myself. It makes me think that they don't really care about me; they just want to have someone that they can go drinking with.

The next step is to identify the potential negative outcomes that may arise if you do not solve this problem:

- I know that my drinking is bad for my long-term health. I don't want to end up with a serious condition a few years down the line.
- When I drink too much I am unpleasant to be around and I don't want to push away the people that I care about.
- I know that I spend way too much money on alcohol that I could be putting towards more important things.

To put it another way, the risks, harms or pain of maintaining the problem need to outweigh the difficulty, discomfort and effort required to solve it.

Once you have committed to solving the problem, make a list of the ways that it could be achieved. In this example:

- Talk to the friend.
- Avoid making plans with the friend by making excuses.
- Avoid them entirely.

You will notice that only one of these options fulfils the criteria of solving the problem while also demonstrating respect to yourself and others. Time to stop biting your tongue and, instead, bite the bullet and call your friend.

Change Your Perception

Sometimes the biggest contributor to a problem is your attitude towards it. Imagine there is someone in your office who has a very irritating laugh. Every time they laugh you think, 'Oh my God, there they go again! Why do they laugh like that?' In no time you have created unnecessary stress for yourself. Rationally you know that they can't help it, and it's not really distracting, you just *don't like it*. In this kind of situation, I'm afraid to say, you may be creating a problem for yourself. Changing your perception would require you to say to yourself something like:

- It's actually really nice to have a cheerful person in the office.
- I really admire that they are confident enough in themselves to not feel self-conscious.
- I wouldn't want to be the person who makes them feel self-conscious about something as healthy as laughing.
- I'm sure plenty of people put up with my foibles, and I'm grateful for that.

This shift in perception reduces the amount of judgement attached to a low-level problem or any situation in which the problem is your attitude and not the behaviour itself.

Learn to Tolerate the Problem

Radical acceptance has its roots in the Buddhist principle of detachment. This does not mean not caring about people or being aloof. Detachment in this sense means letting go of expectation and not overinvesting your emotions in outcomes that are ultimately out of your control.

The idea is that one of the greatest sources of suffering in life comes when things do not go the way we wanted or expected them to go. Some pain is an inevitable part of life. Sometimes people hurt us, or terrible things happen that are completely out of our control. There is nothing we can do about this. Sometimes life is genuinely unfair. However, self-criticism and wishing that things were different, for example refusing to accept reality, can add suffering to the burden of the pain you are already carrying.

I want to be careful here. I am not suggesting that you should just blithely ignore when bad things happen or pretend that you are unaffected. That's not realistic. But I would like you to understand the difference between when you are dealing with the pain and when you are creating suffering. Please see the examples in the box opposite. Hopefully what you notice is that the radical acceptance response still acknowledges the pain (and it may be that significant pain takes a little while to work through), but it does not heap additional suffering on top of that pain.

When you are overly invested in outcomes that are out of your control you put your emotional well-being at the whim of a chaotic and unpredictable universe.

Someone who practises detachment holds the outcome of their efforts or an event very lightly, if at all. Radical acceptance doesn't say you should *like* the situation or think that it is a good thing. What is says is that fighting reality or trying to wish it away creates additional suffering on top of an already painful situation.

Radical acceptance is a powerful intervention for dealing with pain and distressing events, but it is not easy. It takes practice and needs to be applied with subtlety and nuance to each situation.*

* There are, of course, occasions when it would be totally inappropriate and harmful to tolerate or accept a situation. If you are in an abusive environment it would not be right for you to find a way to tolerate it. In all of these situations, your safety is the priority.

Radical acceptance in action

Scenario	Attached response	Radical acceptance	Gratitude bonus
You've had a long day at work and you've never been more ready for your bed. You arrive at the train station to discover that not only have you missed your train, but the one after that is cancelled. You'll have to wait an hour for the next available train.	What? Why? Oh, this is just typical! What am I paying these extortionate ticket prices for? This is ridiculous! Now I'm going to be exhausted tomorrow. Why does this always happen to me?	That's annoying [you're still entitled to acknowledge emotional reality]. Well, I guess there's nothing I can do about it. I can't magic up a train. These things are bound to happen from time to time. So either I wait or I get a taxi. If I wait maybe I can at least catch up on some reading or get ahead on my emails.	At least I will be in my bed at some point. It's not as if I'm going to be here forever. I guess I am lucky that this is the worst thing that has happened to me today.
Your partner decides to end your relationship. You talk it over but they are very clear that, though they care about you, they no longer want to stay together.	Why? Why did it happen? What is it about me? What could I have done differently? Will I ever have another relationship? Maybe I will be alone forever. What happens then? I'm so embarrassed. If they start seeing someone else it means that I meant nothing to them . . .	This. Is. The. Worst. I feel awful. But if they don't want to be with me I can't make them stay. And that would be horrible. I wouldn't want someone to be with me out of obligation. I'm really sad but I suppose this is what happens. Sometimes relationships end.	I am really grateful for the good times that we did have together. Those experiences don't lose their meaning because we are no longer a couple.

Stay Miserable

Psychologist Marsha Linehan does not pull her punches with this option, and deliberately so as it is intended to help individuals to face the often stark reality of their situation, and the way that we all sometimes contribute to our own unhappiness. 'Stay miserable' is really a reminder that if you choose not to apply any of the other techniques to the problem then you are, in some way, choosing to remain unhappy in your current situation. Sure, sometimes we all have a bit of a mope. Feeling sorry for yourself from time to time is normal. In fact, connecting with your pain in this way can help to remind you of why it is so important to do something to change your circumstances in the long-term. But it is not healthy to stay in misery if you can help it.

In my experience, though, saying that someone is choosing to stay miserable isn't quite right or fair. Some people really have tried everything they knew to do. They have tried their best, and nothing improved. These people feel exhausted of hope. I think this is particularly the case for people with the most traumatic backgrounds and especially if the main source of that pain was the immediate family. People who have been abused or left unprotected by their families understandably come to believe that the world is unsafe. If your own family did not love you, then why would anyone else?

I met many women like this when I worked in prison. Women who, as children, had been abused, exploited and neglected by their own parents. When I met with them they often laughed at the idea that life could be better for them. In fact, for many, prison was the safest place they had ever known. Of course, not everyone who has these experiences ends up in prison, and in my clinic I regularly meet people who have what I would call a 'forensic-type history' – the kinds of experiences that led others down a visibly self-destructive route. I say 'visibly' because, though patients in this second group never publicly transgress*, the destructiveness is often internalised, leaving their lives steeped in self-hatred and punishing self-criticism.

I think it is unfair to suggest that these people are 'choosing' to stay miserable, but they certainly develop a negativity bias as a result of the chronic fear and stress of their early life experiences. It can be difficult for such individuals to believe that the road to recovery from harmful relationships comes in the form of more relationships but, of course, healthy ones. They often feel safest not risking depending on anyone but themselves. But, whether it is in finding a loving partner, a genuine friend or the consistent experience of 'kindness and sanity'† that is the core of therapy, it is, I believe, only through experiencing healthy, healing relationships that people with such experiences can reorient their world view to the idea of a world where kindness, love and belonging not only exist, but are available to them.

---

* Often the opposite – abused children often internalise a sense of being 'broken', 'wrong' or 'damaged goods' and compensate for this feeling by creating a façade of perfection and high achievement.
† A description of therapy from philosopher and author Alain de Botton that I particularly like.

It can get better

I met Eve*, a woman in her twenties, when she was referred by the prison officers on her wing who were concerned about her mental state. Eve was recently convicted of a serious violent assault and sentenced to three years in prison. She lost custody of her child and was only granted 'letterbox access', which meant letters and cards were prescreened by social workers. During therapy Eve described a childhood of both violent abuse and extreme neglect that was missed by teachers, medical professionals and social services. Now in prison she told me, 'I know I was put on this earth to suffer.' Week after week Eve told me that there was no point in therapy, she was too broken, I was wasting my time. Week after week I returned to her wing to work with her, even when she told me I was the last person she wanted to see. Yet, whenever I went to her cell to find her, she was waiting for me and so we persisted.

A few months into therapy Eve, whose feelings towards me had moved from outright disdain to mild tolerance, became deeply depressed and suicidal. She told me that she had nothing to live for and that, other than me, no one cared about her. What she could not recognise at the time was that knowing that I cared about her was a sign of hope. If I could care about her, maybe she was someone worth caring about.

We continued the therapy and gradually Eve began to be more engaged with prison life. She got a job in the prison and

* Name has been changed.

took pride in her work. She took educational and skills courses and was praised by her tutors. Each of these actions, these moments of reinforcement, was like a grain of sand in the jar of her self-esteem. We worked together for a little over a year before the decision was made that she was safe enough to move to a lower-security prison. As we worked towards the end of the therapy we reflected on the course of the last year and how she had changed.

'I was a right shit to you.'

I think I might have half-smiled in recognition of the truth in this statement.

'But you never retaliated. That meant everything to me.'

A year or two later I heard news from a colleague who worked in the probation service that on release from prison Eve had started her own business and was applying to college. She was (re)building her life.

Not all people with this set of negative experiences will have such positive outcomes. However, I think Eve's story is a powerful example of how the harm that is done to us in damaging relationships can be repaired in appropriate healthy relationship(s). (It is also, I believe, an illustration of the value of psychotherapeutic interventions in forensic settings.)

Takeaways

- Problems can often feel ambiguous and overwhelming. Understanding what kind of problem(s) you are facing is the first step in getting to grips with it and reminding yourself that you do have some control over the situation or how you manage it.

- Just this step can reduce the amount of stress the problem causes and this is valuable because stress is a major risk to brain health and mental well-being.
- The Four Options are a useful framework for clarifying how to approach a problem. Use them to work through potential strategies before choosing the most appropriate one for you at the time.

CHAPTER 17

How Therapy Can Help

It should come as absolutely no surprise that I, someone who has committed my professional life to providing psychological therapy, would think that therapy is a pretty good thing. However, like any health intervention it comes with the standard caveats: you should find a qualified, experienced and ethical practitioner with whom you feel safe. For therapy to be successful it also needs to be undertaken voluntarily and at the right time. Treatment that comes with external pressure or a time limit rarely ends in a positive or sustainable outcome.

Back in my law firm days as a trainee psychologist I shared an office with a woman who can only fairly be described as a bully. While she didn't take out her misery on me (we were in different departments) she would micromanage, criticise and talk about a woman who worked under her. However, one day she asked me what I was studying:

Me: 'Psychology.'
Her: 'Okay. And what are you going to do with that? Become a counsellor?'
Me: 'Yeah, basically.'
Her: 'Sorry, but I don't see the point in that. I think people

should be able to deal with their problems by themselves. My dad always taught me to be independent.'

Ironically and completely unbeknown to her, she had managed to cram the content of several weeks of therapy into three sentences.

These mistaken beliefs about the nature of the mind, mental health and therapy persist. On an individual level perhaps they don't have much of an impact. Maybe this woman will manage to get through her life without needing to consult a mental health expert. But, unfortunately, her beliefs do not stop with her; if she has children this will be the message that she passes on to them (as her father did to her) and this could make a child who is in a mental health crisis reluctant to reach out for help because to do so would be a sign of 'failure'. We need to address these misperceptions head-on.

I have already made the case that when something goes wrong with an organ or a system we recognise the problem by looking at changes in the *function* of that organ or system. Your brain's *functions* include areas of cognition, perception, personality and mood. It is up to your brain to help you to make decisions efficiently, to hold on to and recall information, to respond appropriately to good news, bad news and humour. So, if you feel persistently sad when the objective conditions of your life are generally okay, or you feel paralysed with anxiety when you need to make a decision, or the idea of seeing your friends starts to fill you with panic, we can deduce that something is wrong. This is the fundamental decision-making process that needs to happen: 'Is my brain functioning the way it usually does when I know I am well?' No. 'Okay, in that case something is up and, considering how important my brain is, I should probably see to that as soon as possible so that it doesn't get worse.'

Unfortunately, in response to the first signs of psychological distress or illness, people are likely to withdraw into isolation, deny what they are experiencing and try to 'push through'. Attitudes similar to the one I described earlier play a large part in why people are reluctant to disclose that they are suffering psychologically – the risk of judgement as 'weak' or 'inadequate' constitutes another source of stress that the person would rather avoid. And I completely understand this. But to the people still operating under the misapprehension that mental illness is a sign of failure, I hope that, having read this far, you now appreciate that mental illnesses are biological disorders deserving of the same care and compassion as other physical ailments.

To anyone who has perhaps held back from seeking help for fear of the reaction of others, please know that there is help out there and you owe it to yourself to ask for your fair share.

What Therapy Is

Therapy is non-invasive brain surgery. In Chapter 13 we saw how 'cells that fire together, wire together'. That is, the more a thought, belief or behaviour is repeated, the greater the reinforcement of those neural networks and the more automatic those processes become. When you first learned to walk, initially coordinating all of those movements took a lot of concentration and repetition. Eventually, this attention reinforced the encoding of the behaviour so that it became unconscious and automatic – you could do it without thinking.

Many forms of psychological distress can be thought of as the automatic pattern of a brain that has been hardwired in a detrimental way. The task of therapy is to reduce the reinforcement of those negative patterns and help clients to hardwire healthier ways of being.

A meta-analysis published in 2018 showed that therapy changes the *physical structure* of the brain. In this analysis the researchers looked at depression, and reviewed studies in which people with depression had had their brains scanned while looking at emotion-provoking images (like a dog baring its teeth). Treatments varied between 11 weeks and 15 months. After therapy (CBT, psychodynamic psychotherapy or interpersonal therapy) there was less activity in the prefrontal cortex, the 'executive' in the brain, which deals with decision-making, planning, social interaction and goal-oriented behaviour. Often in depression there can be too much activity in this area as people catastrophise, playing out the worst-case scenario over and over, and feel others are judging them.

They also found evidence of decreased activity in the cingulate cortex, which is involved in emotion processing and memory and decreased activity in the amygdala. Reduced activation in these areas was interpreted as indicating improved management of fearful or anxiety-provoking stimuli. There was also a significant relationship between treatment and connectivity in areas that help us to suppress the messages from the amygdala, helping us to control our anxiety and not feel overwhelmed by fear and negative thoughts.

People can often feel dubious about therapy. Sometimes it can seem like weird magic. We're not used to the idea that something that isn't medication or a physical intervention can be effective. I hope research like this (and the meditation trials) helps to reassure you (or people who tell you you're wasting your time) that therapy is legit.

What Therapy Is Not

The necessary privacy, and the unnecessary stigma, that surrounds psychological therapy means that few people feel comfortable talking about it. In the vacuum of normal, everyday conversation all sorts of misconceptions, outdated ideas and speculation emerge. I have seen mistaken beliefs about what therapy is get in the way at the start of treatment and I worry that some people who would benefit from a confidential space in which to think about their lives are put off altogether. So I will take this opportunity to bust some myths about therapy:

Your therapist is not only interested in trauma

'But nothing bad happened to me,' is not an uncommon concern raised in an initial therapy session. The popular portrayal of therapy in the media is that it is an intervention people turn to only in cases of severe trauma or crisis. While, of course, counsellors and psychologists are trained to help clients to recover from trauma, much of our work is taken up with the task of helping our patients to *live well*. This means working on self-esteem, relationship issues, major life decisions and adjustment to significant changes, as well as working with psychological illness. At its core therapy is about meaning; trying to understand the 'whys' of life. Why do you have trouble making decisions? Why do you feel tempted to have an affair and what does that mean about your relationship? Why do you feel dissatisfied? None of these questions necessitates a major trauma, but all of them could benefit from being talked through with an impartial, non-judgemental professional.

Therapy is not about blaming everyone else for your problems

'I don't just want to blame my parents for everything. I have to take responsibility for myself.' Another barrier to therapy is the mistaken belief that you and your therapist will collude to try to find ways in which all of the difficulties that you experience can be blamed on somebody else. That approach would actually be counterproductive as it would characterise patients as helpless victims of circumstance who are powerless to affect change in their lives. This would undermine resilience.

Rather, therapy is about reality, and while in reality it is often the case that many of the destructive patterns that we repeat in our lives have their roots in previous significant relationships (whether with parents, siblings, partners or friends), what is also true is that there will be psychological habits and attitudes that you hold that contribute to the maintenance of these difficulties, and it is your therapist's responsibility to draw your attention to these behaviours too.

Therapy is not a soft touch

This one is so wrong it almost makes me laugh. Many people believe that a therapy session is just somewhere that you go to be told what a nice person you are. Though your therapist should always be a kind, safe person for you talk to, that is not the same thing as being permissive.

We are all very good at hiding from ourselves, at turning away from the unpleasant or undesirable aspects of our personalities. We ignore the ways that we might treat others (and ourselves) badly. We all have things that we do or think that we feel deeply ashamed about. Therapy is designed to draw your attention to these unappealing parts of yourself so that you can understand and perhaps change them. For this reason, real therapy, good therapy, is challenging, exhausting, and sometimes excruciating work. But it provides the opportunity for you to break destructive cycles that may have been repeated for generations within a family or many years in your own life. It is hard work, but it is worth it.

Therapy is not going to take over your life

I sometimes wonder whether this one is actually a secret anxiety about how much therapy the person thinks they *need* but, no, your therapist does not want you to stay in treatment for the rest of your life. Speaking personally, one of the most satisfying features of my work is seeing someone develop the confidence, self-belief and skills to start making positive changes in their life. It is an incredible privilege to watch someone's life open up and become more fulfilling. The goal of therapy is to help you live your life, not to replace it.

Therapy is not just talking

Honestly? Psychologists train for at least six years in order to practice. That training includes (amongst other things) neuroanatomy and neuroscience, evolutionary psychology, child development, several theories of personality development across the lifespan, social behaviour, systems psychology, practical clinical skills, risk assessment, psychopathology, research and supervision.

Social support from friends and family is undeniably important in helping to maintain well-being. However, mental health professionals are specially trained to understand, diagnose and treat a range of different psychological issues in evidence-based and effective ways.

Therapy is not only for wealthy, white people

It is important to be honest about some of the class and social obstacles to accessing mental health treatment. In the UK psychological therapy was born out of the psychoanalytic tradition. Psychoanalysis is an intensive approach to personality change and patients attend analysis three to five times per week. Even now, that means that really only very wealthy people who can afford the time and fees can consider undertaking analysis. Since then, many more pragmatic and philosophically diverse forms of therapy have been developed, tested and disseminated and most patients will meet with their therapist once a week. Many therapists will also offer reduced session fees to people on lower incomes.

There is often a cultural reluctance to engage with therapy for people from Black, Asian and Minority Ethnic (BAME) backgrounds. And there are real reasons why BAME people should feel wary of mental health professionals, because racism exists in these organisations.

The Royal College of Psychiatrists (RCP) recognises that black people are grossly overrepresented in the mental health system with both higher overall rates of diagnosis and more severe diagnoses. A black man is 17 times more likely to be diagnosed with a serious mental health disorder than a white man. The RCP says that racism is a key reason for this disparity, noting: 'racism and racial discrimination can have a significant, negative impact on a person's life chances and mental health . . . it can lead to a profound feeling of pain, harm and humiliation, often leading to despair and exclusion'. Unconscious bias in the attending professionals also plays a part. A study published in 2017 found that people perceive black men as larger and more threatening than same-sized white men. They are then more likely to be targeted by police and more likely to endure physical restraint and arrest (instead of hospitalisation) when in acute mental distress.

Mental illness is also highly stigmatised in many BAME cultures, being considered a source of further shame in an environment in which BAME individuals and communities are already looked down upon, or a sign of moral or spiritual failure. The cruel irony is that it is often the experiences of marginalisation and prejudice that contribute to the erosion of mental well-being that drive the need for psychotherapeutic intervention.

It is also true that psychology and psychological therapy teams are predominately composed of white, middle-class practitioners. This relative underrepresentation of BAME practitioners, especially in the context of the disproportionate number of BAME patients, is something that the professional organisations are trying to understand. BAME clients often find it easier to open up to professionals whom they feel already understand aspects of their culture or lived experience, and where issues of race and identity can be discussed without fear of upsetting their therapist. I have supplied a list of counselling services accustomed to dealing with race-related distress on page 317.

Therapy is not homophobic

I would like to dispel another myth, or rather an antiquated idea, that perhaps some people worry still exists in the field. Homosexuality is not seen as a mental illness or a lifestyle choice. No ethical practitioner will ever try to 'make someone straight' and so-called 'conversion therapy' has been roundly condemned by all of the UK's major therapy regulatory bodies, including the British Psychological Society, the British Psychoanalytic Council and the UK Council for Psychotherapy.

Protecting the Mental Health of Future Generations

It is true that each person finds their way to therapy for a unique and important reason. It would be a gross oversimplification to say that the emotional or psychological difficulties that a person faces in adulthood can always be traced back to some childhood difficulty. Adult trauma, work stress, bereavement and grief, relationship issues, infidelity, and existential threats such as illness and mortality are pressing dilemmas that deserve the time and thoughtful attention offered by counselling and therapy. Yet, mental health and social care professionals are in unanimous agreement that the developmentally sensitive period of the early years and childhood are critical in giving a child the best opportunity and resources to develop into an emotionally resilient adult. No, there is no fool-proof system; when it comes to personality development and psychological health some people manage to do well with very little, while others whom we might think of as having been very privileged may struggle. In this way psychological distress does not discriminate. However, there are known factors and events in early life that increase an individual's risk of mental ill health in adulthood that I believe all responsible parents should be aware of.

To be unsparingly honest, I write this on behalf of the many clients over my years of clinical practice who have fought coura-geously to reclaim their lives and their self-esteem following decades of confusion and self-doubt. People who have held back from exploring their full potential because they believed them-selves to be unworthy or insignificant. I fully acknowledge that I, by the very nature of my work, see a very particular sample of the population, but it is also true that very many people suffer who do not seek the help they deserve. I also acknowledge that, so often, the parents who emotionally harm their children were also victims of similar harms themselves. What I say is not meant as a condem-nation, but comes bound in a deep compassion for anyone who has worked to undo the damage that was done to them as a child.

Address your own pain first

It is by no means inevitable that someone who had a neglectful or abusive parent in childhood will present similar harm to their own children. But pain that has not been addressed has a way of re-emerg-ing at key moments in our lives. Perhaps not in the same form; maybe as grief, or depression, or envy (strange as it may seem, parents can and do envy their own children). Whatever form it takes, this unresolved pain can interfere with a parent's capacity to care for their own child. It is as if there are 'ghosts in the nursery' and the parent can be so preoccupied with trying to expel these ghosts that their attention is taken away from the current needs of the child(ren).

If you know that you have had a 'difficult' experience or relationship with one or both of your parents, please consider working with a professional to resolve this before starting a family.

Having a baby won't fix your relationship

Facing the end of a long and meaningful relationship can be unbearable. When a partnership that was once so nourishing hits the rocks or is already sinking, there can be a wish to deny this reality. We hope that it is a phase or that there is some other way of staving off the inevitable. In these circumstances the responsible thing to do is to seek support for your relationship, to work out what is contributing to the current difficulties and to decide how they can be remedied. Some individuals and couples though, unwilling or unable to face the reality of the potential ending, will hope that the issues will be resolved by having a (or another) child. Not only is this a mistaken hope (a newborn will only add pressure to the existing cracks in the relationship), it is also a misuse of a life. A child is not superglue. Having a child to 'save' a relationship is, by definition, using the baby as a means to an end. It's unfair and destined to fail.

If your relationship is in trouble and you are unsure what to do, resources are provided on page 319.

You create the universe your child sees and lives in

This is really a reminder to not underestimate how much attention your child is paying to you. What you might think of as an innocuous comment becomes part of the representation of the world for your child. Whether it is describing someone on the TV as 'fat and ugly' or laughing at a racist joke, as a parent you have enormous power to create and reinforce not just your own child's self-esteem but also social norms for years to come.

Tough love does not produce emotional resilience
'My dad was tough on me and it didn't do me any harm.' The notion of 'tough love' is a total misunderstanding of what factors promote psychological resilience. Really it is the difference between a brittle toughness and flexible strength; the difference between breaking down under pressure and bouncing back.

To foster durable resilience, children need to know two things:

1. They are fundamentally worthwhile.
2. They are still loved even when they 'mess up' or show emotion.

These are the foundations of a robust self-esteem that will enable the person to recover from mistakes and troubles rather than collapse into castigation and self-loathing. Enforce reasonable boundaries but don't bully your children under the guise of 'tough love'.

Don't make negative comparisons
'Why can't you be more like your clever/thin/etc. cousin/sister/family friend?', 'You're just like your father in that way,' ('that way' being something that you have previously disparaged). Please don't do this.

Don't use your child as a weapon
Hopefully this one doesn't need much explanation. It is, frankly, immoral to use your child to hurt the other parent. Whether it's

trying to turn the child against the other or threatening to deny access, unless the child is in danger, playing these sorts of cruel games ultimately hurts the child the most. Why do I say 'immoral'? Because these behaviours are another example of using the child as a means to an end, as an object with which to hurt the other parent, and treating a child like that, with disregard for his/her needs, is unconscionable.

Don't use your child as a buffer or go-between

This kind of behaviour interferes with the child's opportunity to have a healthy independent relationship with both parents. It also pushes them into a precociously adult position in which they are the mediator between two adults who are neglecting their responsibilities as parents. Again, please see page 319 for resources to address any difficulties in your relationship.

Don't use your child as your therapist

'You're the only one I can talk to.' This is an inappropriate and unfair burden to place on the shoulders of a child. Do what you can to find an adult to talk to so that you are able to be a parent to your child, and not the other way around.

I am of the opinion that becoming a parent should not be considered a right but a privilege and a responsibility. A child is not a possession but a conscious being deserving of dignity, which is to say they have the right to respect and to be treated fairly, for their own sake, not as an extension of the parent(s). This foundation of love and dignity becomes the launch pad from which children have the best opportunity to thrive and grow into independent, compassionate and emotionally resilient adults and citizens.

Know the signs

Children are often unable or frightened to speak up when they are suffering. Knowing the signs of a child who might be at risk may help to protect that child sooner. The list below provides examples of common signs of distress in children. The list is not exhaustive and children with these symptoms may not be being abused or bullied, but they may be struggling emotionally in some other way. The more caring adults who know the signs, the safer children will be.

- Withdrawal, being more quiet than usual
- No longer wanting to do activities they previously enjoyed and other changes in behaviour
- Drop in academic/school performance
- Frequent stomach aches
- Wishing to avoid certain places or people
- Bedwetting, especially in children who have passed that stage of development
- Increased apathy, nervousness, anxiety, aggression or violence
- Tearfulness
- Precocious knowledge – knowing about 'grown up' things too soon
- School truancy, frequent absences or running away
- Dirty clothes or inappropriate dress for the weather conditions
- Unexplained bruises or attempts to cover limbs even in hot weather
- Avoids mealtimes
- Disclosure of difficulty or abuse

It is important to not ignore these signs, even if it is simply to say that you have noticed a change and ask the child if they are okay. If the child makes a disclosure of mistreatment it is important to believe them and act accordingly. There should be no shame in discovering abuse, only in ignoring, denying or covering it up.

Takeaways

- Therapy is a powerful, often challenging psychological intervention that can literally reshape the brain.
- You do not need a history of trauma or to have received a psychiatric diagnosis to benefit from therapy. In the same way that most people wouldn't think twice about going for a physical health check-up or hiring a personal trainer, therapy can be a means of ensuring your brain (the most complex organ in the body) is functioning at its best.
- Parents have enormous power to shape not only how their child grows to view themselves, but what kind of citizen they will be in the world.
- As a parent your responsibility is to do what you can to ensure that your child(ren) grow up believing that they are worthwhile human beings in their own right, not simply for how they look or what they achieve.
- Avoid using your child to fulfil your own emotional needs. It is an inappropriate level of responsibility for a child and risks depriving your child of their dignity.
- Tough love promotes brittle 'hardness', which is not the same as secure resilience. In reality it equates to little more than bullying.

CHAPTER 18

Making Change Stick

The way we conceptualise and treat mental illness is fundamentally flawed. It simply does not make sense to think of the brain and the body as independent systems or to treat them as such. The evidence, as I hope I have conveyed, is clear and compelling: the body and the brain are one system. Attempting to treat psychological distress without also attending to the body and lifestyle severely limits the efficacy of that treatment. Trying to develop new neural pathways in a brain that is under-slept and undernourished is an uphill struggle. It is incumbent on us all – patients, practitioners and policymakers – to start keeping the body in mind when we are thinking about neurological disease and mental illness.

In my clinic I call this approach 'Whole Body Mental Health' and use it as a framework for developing comprehensive and effective treatments for my clients. The team, composed of dieticians, exercise physiologists and psychologists, collaborate to understand the underlying causes of the client's mental health complaints and to identify the areas most amenable to change and improvement.

But we should not be waiting until a person is unwell enough to need treatment. Every other arena of healthcare has adopted a 'prevention first' approach, except mental health. In psychiatry 'early intervention' means the first sign of illness or the first presentation to a GP. This is not prevention. Prevention means helping the public to understand the known risk factors of psychological distress, empowering them to intervene where they can and enacting policy for the social determinants of health. This book is my contribution to the former.

I know I have presented you with a huge range of brain-health-promoting factors and I would not blame you for feeling overwhelmed. I wish I could narrow it down to one simple list of 'Do this, not that,' but health is never that straightforward and it would be disingenuous of me to suggest otherwise. However, this is not a book about brain-health theory; I do want to help you to implement as many of these powerful and practical behaviours into your life, and that means making that process as easy as possible. But, first, we need to address the barriers to change . . . or why you won't take any of the advice in this book!

Barriers to Change

Psychologists study the human mind and behaviour, and one of the most curious things about human beings is how irrational and self-defeating we can be. Even if we start out with the best intentions, we are experts at getting in our own way and that's, in part, because of a long list of thinking errors called 'cognitive biases'. Your brain, as wonderful and clever as it is, is also very busy and wherever possible it likes to save energy. A cognitive bias is a kind of thinking shortcut. We develop them because, a lot of the time, they help to reduce the amount of effort your brain has to go to when making decisions. The problem is that they are easily influenced by irrelevant information while at the same time appearing to be reliable or true.

Cognitive biases can be a big barrier to any kind of change; they have a tendency to emphasise the difficulties and minimise the benefits of trying something new. I want to give you all the very best chances of implementing the tips and tools in this book. Therefore, for the sake of transparency and to hopefully give you an advantage over your own psychology, here is a summary of some of the cognitive biases and other irrational thinking behaviours that might get in the way of you making the small but important changes required to help improve your long-term brain health.

'But I'm young now' (delay discounting or future discounting)
This is going to be the big one. We all have an innate preference for things that will pay off in the short-term over things we can look forward to in the future. For example, if I were to offer you £5 right now or £10 in two weeks, the vast majority of people would take the £5, even though they would be better off waiting. We do this ALL THE TIME.

On top of this we live in a media environment in which we are always being offered the next 'quick fix' for our health or lifestyle problems, whether it's a 12-week 'body blitz', waist trainers, superfoods or a new miracle exercise regime. Commercial diet plans make a big deal of how quickly you can expect weight loss, even if that loss is unrealistic and unsustainable; 'quick loss now' is significantly more appealing than 'slow loss over several months'. This makes it very hard for us to hold in mind and value something that seems a long way off.

When it comes to taking care of your brain, I can't promise you immediate 'results'. For example, most Alzheimer's disease is diagnosed in your sixties, but the damage to the brain is visible in brain scans during your forties. The brain can compensate for small amounts of damage for a while, which means it takes several years before accumulated lesions show up as recognisable signs and symptoms, by which point the damage is largely irreversible.

People should start to take their brain health seriously from at least middle age (ideally earlier), but most won't see the benefits for a further two decades, meaning the value of the future payoff feels much lower than the cost of the effort right now. But, when it comes to brain health, it's all about playing the long game.

'It won't happen to me' (optimism bias and denial)

This one sounds positive but it can be a real problem when it comes to getting people to change their behaviours or to take certain health risks seriously. We assume that the rules or risks that apply to the rest of the world do not apply to ourselves. Classically, smokers recognise that smoking causes lung cancer but individual smokers believe that they *themselves* are at no increased risk of the disease.

Part of this effect is explained by our tendency to want to avoid thinking about painful or unpleasant things. No one wants to imagine themselves (or their loved ones) in poor health or dying. So we turn a blind eye to the real-life risks of our harmful habits or, even worse, ignore the early warning signs of illness. How often after a catastrophe do we lament not heeding the warning? Denial is a hugely powerful psychological state that, as a psychologist, I encounter regularly in my clients when things are simply too painful to think about. What I have to help them to understand is that the long-term danger of avoiding this unpleasant aspect of reality outweighs the immediate pain of doing so. When we can agree on that then I can help them to engage in facing whatever painful reality they are grappling with.

While I think it is great to be optimistic about one's health, it is also important not to take it for granted, and that means doing what you can when you can to help protect your brain health and mental well-being. Try not to think of a new health habit as a chore but as an opportunity to invest in yourself and in your future.

'My grandmother lived to be 102 and she was absolutely fine' (anchoring bias)

This one is similar to the optimism bias but it relies on a single piece of 'evidence' as proof, and it is even more powerful if the example feels close to home. Even if the research tells us that there are certain habits that have been reliably shown to improve brain health and mental wellness, and even if we know we aren't doing them, having ready access to the story of a single outlier will give us all the confidence we need to convince ourselves that we will also buck the trend. Instead of thinking that maybe Grandma was just lucky or that there might be any number of other factors influencing her health and longevity that you will never know about, you rely on the example of her health as a sure sign that you will be just fine too, thank you very much.

Again, be optimistic but try not to take your health for granted.

'But change is really hard' (status quo bias)

This attitude is the final nail in the coffin for so many attempts to make behavioural or lifestyle changes. You can also think about it as a fear of change. Sometimes it doesn't matter how convinced we are of the potential benefits of change, we all get used to the way things are and how they have always been. In fact, sometimes we get so locked into our habits that we forget that we have a choice to alter things and that change is possible. In clinic I often see people who feel compelled to stay as they are, even if it is uncomfortable, because it is familiar. It is as though they have been treading the same path for so long that it has become a trench that they can no longer see out of.

It is true that change takes effort; our everyday ways of thinking and behaving become habitual and automatic (though we forget that even these familiar behaviours were once new to us). But equally, change and adaptation are hallmarks of our species. Our ability to learn new skills and adjust to new environments is the reason that we have been able to adapt to live in almost any conditions on the planet. You have to remember that this capacity to change continues to exist in you.

The problem is, we tend to see change in 'all-or-nothing' terms. Win or lose. Pass or fail. This is not actually how it works. Take a look at the 'cycle of change' diagram on the next page. Change is a process. First, we have to become aware of our current habits. Then we have to make a plan of how to introduce new ones. After that we must recognise all the moments when we slip back into our old ways. This slipping back can be a real challenge because, if you take a harsh all-or-nothing view, it feels more like failure than the inevitable and encouraging signs of change. This frustration can lead the majority of people to give up before they start to really enjoy the benefits of their efforts.

The cycle of change

People often don't realise that change isn't just something that you do. For most of us adopting new behaviours isn't a switch that you turn on and off, it is a process that you enter into. The cycle of change looks like this:

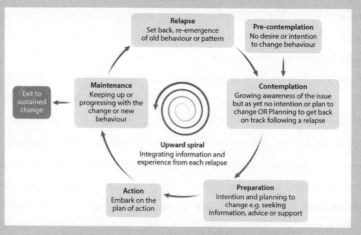

Adapted from Prochaska and Diclemente (1986)

If we take quitting smoking as an example of a health-promoting behavioural change, the individual stages might take the following form:

1. Pre-contemplation: 'I'm a smoker. I haven't even considered not smoking. It's just something I do. I enjoy it. Excuse me, I'm just popping out for a cigarette.'
2. Contemplation: 'Huh. So I just read about the effects that smoking might be having on my health. I do find I struggle to catch my breath when I work out. Maybe it's not great for me. But let's not make any rash decisions.'

3. Preparation: 'All right, I'm going to stop. I've looked up all the tips and asked my friends who have stopped what worked for them.'

4. Action: Depending on which rotation of the upward cycle the person is on this might be anything from making a plan, purchasing nicotine patches, reducing the number of daily cigarettes or switching to e-cigarettes, for example.

5. Maintenance: 'Great! I smoked one less cigarette today than usual. Let's see if I can do the same tomorrow.'

6. Relapse: 'Damn! I smoked loads last night. I had been doing so well.'

What's that? Relapse is part of the cycle of change? Yes! The problem is that, when trying to implement a new behaviour or break an old habit, most people look at the process in absolute terms: either I am winning or I am failing completely. This black-and-white thinking means that when they eventually relapse, rather than seeing it as an inevitable part of the process, cutting themselves some slack and moving on to the next rotation of the upward spiral, they think they have failed, which puts them at risk of giving up trying altogether.

Please remember this as you start the process of building your brain-healthy lifestyle. There will be times when you forget or fall back and this is totally to be expected. This is what change looks like.

'Out of sight, out of mind'

Your poor brain is really up against it in the fight for recognition. Not least of all because you can't see it. This is the challenge I have tried to get to grips with when trying to help people to think about their brains on social media, the ground zero for diet plans and exercise programmes for the body. You don't have to go far on Instagram to come across a 'body transformation' plan. These programmes (in line with most weight loss diets) enjoy popularity because the rapidity with which they create a (wholly unsustainable) calorie deficit means that dieters will start to see 'results' very quickly. This swift feedback reinforces feelings of agency ('I can do it') and efficacy ('It's working') that help people to stick with the plan.

Now, let's compare that to the situation for your brain. Locked away behind your skull, it isn't possible to take a quick peak at your brain 'gains'. There is no visual comparison to keep you motivated. Along with delay discounting this means that not only are you not likely to be thinking about what's going on in your brain (until something starts to go wrong), even when you do, the risks are likely to feel way off in the future and not worth thinking about right now.

You can try to reduce the impact of this bias by keeping track of your moods. Rate your mood between 1 and 10 (1 is 'very poor' and 10 is 'great') at the start of every week (you can do this as part of your 'start the week' practice – page 201). Hopefully, over time you will see an improvement in your moods, mental clarity and energy, which are all good signs that your brain is benefiting from the changes.

You may also find it helpful to know that a 'multi-domain' approach – that focuses on several lifestyle habits rather than a single magic bullet – like the one outlined in this book has already been shown to improve brain health. The Finnish Geriatric Intervention Study to Prevent Cognitive Impairment and Disability (FINGER) supported older people with a high risk of dementia to improve nutrition, physical activity, cognitive training (staying mentally engaged) and social activity. After two years they found that maintaining a brain-healthy lifestyle could preserve and even *improve* cognitive function. This is brilliant news, especially since we still seem to be a long way away from effective medications. Prevention works!

Overcoming Barriers to Change

I know that changing your habits and behaviours is really difficult. Not only is it daunting at the outset, but the inevitable relapses can be demoralising and tempt you to quit altogether. Making change stick requires a few elements to be in place:

- A compelling, intrinsic reason: You need to have a strong, personal reason why you want to make these changes. The Future Self exercise (page 302) is designed to tackle future discounting and optimism bias by getting you to contemplate what it will feel like to be you in a few years. In effect I will be sending you into the future. By making the future more proximate I hope to be able to help you recognise the value of investing for it in the present.
- A clear plan with attainable goals: A plan is the essential roadmap for change. Your plan tells you in which direction you are heading, tracked by milestones that you hit along the way.
- Ease of implementation: Remember, your brain will take shortcuts wherever it can. Knowing this means that your plan needs to accommodate for this tendency. It's not good enough for it to work when you are feeling your best; the plan needs to be easy to stick to when you are tired, cranky and unmotivated.
- Self-compassion: If you need to make significant changes it is *inevitable* that you will 'mess up'. Inevitable. It is important to

have compassion for yourself when this happens; being hard on yourself will only make you feel worse. Remind yourself that this is what change looks like, remind yourself of all the progress you have made and of your motivation. Then find something that gives you a quick win for a much-needed morale boost.

- Commitment devices: These are a way of increasing the downside of not making a change by creating a significant (but not disastrous) penalty for yourself for not complying. An effective one is to tell people what you intend to do. In this way the gentle social pressure of wanting to appear consistent, and not wanting to damage your reputation, can help to keep you on track. Anticipating setbacks and finding ways to mitigate them can also help increase your chances of success.

You may have noticed that I have not listed willpower as one of the requirements of change. Unfortunately, willpower is not reliable enough for you to depend on, especially when you are tired, distracted or under pressure. In these situations, we may simply not have the energy to maintain the levels of willpower required for change. Furthermore, individual personality differences may influence how able we are to draw on willpower, with people who score higher on conscientiousness being more likely than low scorers to resist temptation and maintain focus. So, willpower may give some people an extra boost but, by itself, it is not sufficient for most people to sustain change.

Say hello to your Future Self

We are powerfully biased towards the present; the future feels far away and future outcomes feel only distantly related to what we do today. But in order to take prevention seriously we have to feel some connection and concern for our future welfare. The following exercise is designed to heighten your sense of connection to your Future Self. Try it twice: first as if you close this book and nothing changes, and again imagining you have taken some of the recommended actions. Find somewhere quiet and comfortable to sit and close your eyes.

> Imagine you are sitting at a table in a sunny kitchen. A few moments later you, 10 years from now, walk in and sit opposite you. How do you look? How do you move? What emotions can you read in your face? How do you feel?
>
> What do you want to say to the present-day version of you? What advice do you want to give yourself?

Another way of reminding yourself of just how quickly time passes is to send yourself an email in the future (https://www.futureme.org is a website that allows you to easily send scheduled emails). Write yourself two short emails: schedule one for a week from now and one for a month from today. If you are someone who tends to put things off, this can be a useful exercise to help you keep in mind that 'the future' comes around very quickly. The actions you take to invest in your brain health today will influence the mental health you enjoy tomorrow.

Meaning

Remember that meaning drives motivation and, when we are trying to introduce new behaviours, having a clear sense of meaning can help us to tolerate the effort that comes with change, improving our chances of success.

On the lines below (or on a separate piece of paper) I would like you to complete the following sentences:

- I want to introduce brain-healthy habits into my life because . . .
. . . .
. . . .
- The added benefit to my friends and family will be . . . .
. . . .
. . . .
- If I do not make these changes I am afraid that my future will . . .
. . . .
. . . .
- I will ask . . . . to do it with me.

In the table on the following pages I have broken down the key elements of a brain-healthy lifestyle into quick and easy tasks, many of which can be completed in less than five minutes. Your challenge is to tick off three different tasks per day. Each task must be in a different category, so it's not enough for you to have a salad of spinach, spring onions and beans and be done. That's great (and delicious) but all of those habits are in the same category. But have a handful of nuts (B6), floss before bed (C1) and go for a walk at lunchtime (D1) and you are winning. Try to vary the habits throughout the weeks to introduce a broad range of actions into your repertoire. It may not feel like you are doing very much, but over time these changes accumulate to create an overall brain-healthy lifestyle. You can find a print-friendly version of this form at: kimberleywilson.co/resources.

See how many you tick off at the end of the week and review where you could perhaps introduce another beneficial change.

A		Sleep
	1	Avoided coffee after midday.
	2	Got 30 minutes of natural light in the morning or at lunchtime.
	3	Turned lights down at least an hour before bed.
	4	Stopped using light-emitting devices at least an hour before bed.
	5	Kept the bedroom cool.
	6	Kept the bedroom dark.
	7	Wrote down any worries or tasks for the next day.
	8	Avoided doing work in bed or in the bedroom.
	9	Avoided alcohol in the two hours before bed.
	10	Avoided drinking too much liquid before bed.
B		Food
	1	Ate a serving (small bowlful) of leafy greens.
	2	Ate a cup of berries.
	3	Prepared a meal with three different herbs and/or spices (not including salt and pepper).
	4	Ate a serving of alliums.
	5	Ate half a tin of beans.
	6	Ate a handful of raw nuts.
	7	Had a serving of cold carbs.
	8	Had a serving of wholegrains.
	9	Drank one cup of tea or coffee.
	10	Ate a portion of oily fish.
C		Dental health
	1	Flossed at least once today.
	2	Brushed teeth in the morning and evening.
	3	Booked a check-up with the dentist.

D		Physical activity and exercise
	1	Walked for at least 10 minutes.
	2	Exercised vigorously for 20 minutes.
	3	Moderately exercised for 30 minutes.
	4	Did strength training of a major muscle group (legs, hips, back, abdomen, chest, shoulders and arms).
	5	Did 30 minutes of mindful movement such as yoga or stretching.
	6	Got up every 50 minutes for a walk/stretch.
E		Breath
	1	Did at least two minutes of slow, controlled breathing.
	2	Sang a power ballad in the shower.
	3	Attended a yoga or other mindful movement class.
F		Heat
	1	Spent 20 minutes in the sauna or a hot bath.
G		Attention
	1	Did 20 minutes of mindfulness practice.
	2	Did 20 minutes of learning.
	3	Read uninterrupted for 20 minutes.
H		Critical thinking
	1	Applied CT questions to a claim read on social media.
I		Social media and tech
	1	Put phone away when trying to work.
	2	Put phone away when talking to my partner or a friend.
J		Money
	1	Checked my bank account.
	2	Drafted a budget.

K		Emotions
	1	Wrote down how I am feeling and thought about why.
	2	Talked to a friend about what is bothering me.
	3	Went to therapy.
	4	Watched 20 minutes of comedy.
L		Relationships
	1	Called a friend or family member for a catch-up.
	2	Made a plan to meet up with a friend(s) in the next two weeks.
	3	Attended an interactive group activity such as a book club.
	4	Put phone away when talking to friends and family face-to-face.
	5	Let someone know they can call me if they need to talk.

If you go to kimberleywilson.co/resources you can find a number of self-measure questionnaires that you can use to track changes in your mood and quality of life, which, while not as accurate as a brain scan, will provide some insight into your well-being.

Finally, I would love you to join the community of allstars who are beating the odds by implementing these changes on the Healthy Brain Instagram and Facebook groups. If you do, you will be giving your chances an extra boost by seeing examples of other people like you who are doing it and who are keeping each other accountable with tips and encouragement.

Are You a Policymaker?

The limits of lifestyle

Throughout this book I have tried to make the case for how important lifestyle, thinking and relational behaviours are in promoting emotional well-being and helping to protect your brain health for the long-term. I hope I have convinced you that there are numerous opportunities throughout your day to make small changes that, collectively, equate to important brain-health improvements.

However, it would be unfair (and, I think, unethical) of me to leave you with the impression that all the power is solely in your hands because there are real limits to what lifestyle changes can do for us.

The 'social determinants of health' are the characteristics of our lives and living environments that impact our health but are beyond our control. These include:

- In utero exposure: your genetics and the hormones, medications, bacteria, nutrients, etc. you were exposed to during pregnancy.
- Birth trauma.

- Adverse childhood experiences: chronic stressful events during childhood, such as witnessing or experiencing domestic violence, neglect or abuse, maternal and parental mental illness, family instability, having a parent in prison, growing up in poverty or with an addicted parent, all leave a biological scar on the child that can persist into adulthood, increasing their risk of psychological difficulties.
- Quality of available schooling.
- Access to green space and fresh air in your neighbourhood.
- Safety and accessibility of active commuting options.
- Membership of a marginalised group: people of minority groups often experience overt prejudice or covert limitations on their opportunities for success and career progression, factors that constitute chronic stressors that undermine mental health.
- Income and working conditions.
- Quality of and access to local healthcare.
- Availability of social support.
- Levels of social equality in your community.

This is a long and daunting list, but it should not make us feel that it is futile to make the important changes outlined in this book. What it should do is encourage us to demand more from our elected officials and policymakers.

It is in every government's best interests to have a happy, healthy population.

However, one of the many things that health professionals of all disciplines must be careful of is the risk of making individuals responsible for the harms that have been done to them by society.

The life expectancy in Scotland is approximately two years shorter than it is in England. Even more strikingly, the life expectancy between cities in the same country can vary dramatically. A man born in the outer-Glasgow district of East Dunbartonshire will live *seven years* longer than if he was born and raised in Glasgow city. Poverty, food deserts, poor healthcare provision, school class size, local employment opportunities, air pollution, access to green spaces, crime and quality of housing are among the many factors outside of the individual's scope of influence, which will have a direct impact on health. It is disingenuous and a dereliction of duty to place the full burden of health responsibility on the individual.

Instead, it is proper that we turn to policymakers at local, national and international level to demonstrate their commitment to true parity between physical and mental health. Neurological and psychiatric disorders confer some of the heaviest burdens of disease and disability of any health condition. The burden is felt not only by the individual patient but their children, carers, employers and health services.

If you have read this far, then I will presume that you value this information personally or for your family. However, as someone in a position of policy authority it is incumbent upon you to campaign for the needs of the people you represent. People whose circumstances at birth put them at a quantifiable health disadvantage.

Since the risks and harms outlined are long-term in nature, taking years and often decades to emerge as symptoms, policies must be equally long-standing, focused on early intervention and prevention. Effective policies will require multilevel collaboration and cross-party agreement.

If you're not sure where to start, I fortunately have a list of suggestions:

- Early intervention programmes for pregnant women to optimise maternal health and nutrition (including alcohol and drug services and smoking cessation), and assess any additional psychological support needs.
- Programme of nutritional supplementation for at-risk children for the first 1,000 days of life.
- Increased investment in programmes to support troubled families.
- Inclusion of brain and mental health awareness on high school curricula.
- Investment in programmes to promote and facilitate safe active commuting.
- Review of industry-specific working conditions.
- Provisions to improve air quality, particularly around nurseries, schools, parks and children's play areas.
- Improved regulation of social media influencer marketing.
- A comprehensive public health campaign for the brain.
- Increased investment in clinical research of preventative strategies and treatments for cognitive decline and neurological disorders.
- Pilot a 'dual appointment' in which a psychologist is present during GP consultations.
- Provision of micronutrients to prisoners as this reduces risk of violence.

Only by making a sincere, long-term commitment to improving the brain and mental health of our communities can we hope to reverse the many predicted increases in suicide rates, mental illness diagnoses and neurodegenerative disease.

Basic Rest-Activity Cycle (BRAC) Tracker

Day 1		Day 2		Day 3	
	Interval		Interval		Interval
Average					

The average length of time between yawns was:......................................

My ideal bedtime is: ....

APPENDIX 2

Emulsifiers

E numbers	Additives
E322	Lecithins
E407	Carrageenan
E410	Locust bean gum; carob gum (IBS)
E412	Guar gum (IBS)
E415	Xanthan gum
E417	Tara gum
E418	Gellan gum (Gut)
E433	Polyoxyethylene sorbitan mono-oleate; Polysorbate 80
E466	Carboxy methyl cellulose (CMC)

Resources

Cross-Cultural Therapy Services

BAATN: The Black, African and Asian Therapy Network
www.baatn.org.uk
connect@baatn.org.uk

Muslim Counsellor & Psychotherapist Network
www.mcapn.co.uk
admin@mcapn.co.uk

Nafsiyat: Intercultural Therapy Centre
Unit 4
Lysander Mews
N19 3QP
020 7263 6947
www.nafsiyat.org.uk
admin@nafsiyat.org.uk

Gambling Support Services

BeGambleAware
www.begambleaware.org

GamCare
www.gamcare.org.uk

National Gambling Helpline
24 hours, seven days a week
0808 8020 133

Help Managing Debt

Citizens Advice
www.citizensadvice.org.uk

National Debtline
0808 808 4000
www.nationaldebtline.org

PayPlan
0800 280 2816
www.payplan.com

StepChange
0800 138 1111
www.stepchange.org

The Money Advice Service
0800 138 7777
www.moneyadviceservice.org.uk

Relationship Counselling Services

Relate: The Relationship People
www.relate.org.uk

Online Learning Resources

Art Prof
Free art education platform
artprof.org

Future Learn
Free online courses from top universities
www.futurelearn.com

Institute of Ideas
Online library of over 1,000 talks from the world's leading thinkers
www.iai.tv/debates-and-talks

Khan Academy
Free lessons, practice exercises, instructional videos on a range of
academic subjects
www.khanacademy.org

Open Culture
1,300 free online courses from top universities
www.openculture.com

Project Gutenberg
A library of over 60,000 free eBooks
www.gutenberg.org

References

Introduction

Alzheimer's Research UK, 2019. Dementia attitudes monitor. Retrieved from https://www.dementiastatistics.org/wp-content/uploads/2019/02/Dementia -Attitudes-Monitor-Wave-1-Report.pdf#zoom=100, accessed 16 Feb. 2019.

Brown, D. and Triggle, N., 2018. Mental health: 10 charts on the scale of the problem. *BBC News*. Retrieved from https://www.bbc.co.uk/news/health -41125009, accessed 4 Oct. 2019.

Gesch, C. B., Hammond, S. M., Hampson, S. E., Eves, A. and Crowder, M. J., 2002. Influence of supplementary vitamins, minerals and essential fatty acids on the antisocial behaviour of young adult prisoners: Randomised, placebo-controlled trial. *The British Journal of Psychiatry*, *181*(1), pp.22–8. doi: 10.1192/bjp.181.1.22.

Jacka, F. N., Pasco, J. A., Mykletun, A., Williams, L. J., Hodge, A. M., O'Reilly, S. L., Nicholson, G. C., Kotowicz, M. A. and Berk, M., 2010. Association of Western and traditional diets with depression and anxiety in women. *American Journal of Psychiatry*, *167*(3), pp.305–11. doi: 10.1176/ appi.ajp.2009.09060881.

Livingston, G., Sommerlad, A., Orgeta, V., Costafreda, S. G., Huntley, J., Ames, D., Ballard, C., Banerjee, S., Burns, A., Cohen-Mansfield, J. and Cooper, C., 2017. Dementia prevention, intervention, and care. *The Lancet*, *390*(10113), pp.2673–2734. doi: 10.1016/S0140-6736(17)31363-6.

Loftus, E. F. and Palmer, J. C., 1974. Reconstruction of automobile destruction: An example of the interaction between language and memory. *Journal of Verbal Learning and Verbal Behavior, 13*(5), pp.585–9. doi: 10.1016/S0022-5371(74)80011-3.

Lourida, I., Hannon, E., Littlejohns, T. J., Langa, K. M., Hyppönen, E., Kuźma, E. and Llewellyn, D. J., 2019. Association of lifestyle and genetic risk with incidence of dementia. *JAMA, 322*(5), pp.430–7. doi:10.1001/jama.2019.9879.

Lukianoff, G. & Haidt, J. 2018. *The Coddling of the American Mind: How Good Intentions and Bad Ideas are Setting Up a Generation for Failure.* Allen Lane.

Mohdin, A., 4 Sep. 2018. Suicide rate rises among young people in England and Wales. Retrieved from https://www.theguardian.com/society/2018/sep/04/suicide-rate-rises-among-young-people-in-england-and-wales, accessed 16 Feb. 2019.

NHS, 5 Oct. 2016. Symptoms: clinical depression. Retrieved from https://www.nhs.uk/conditions/clinical-depression/symptoms/, accessed 16 Feb. 2019.

Nomis: Official Labour Market Statistics. Mortality statistics. Retrieved from https://www.nomisweb.co.uk/query/select/getdatasetbytheme.asp?theme=73, accessed 16 Feb. 2019.

Office for National Statistics, 2018. Deaths registered in England and Wales (series DR): 2017. Retrieved from https://www.ons.gov.uk/peoplepopulationandcommunity/birthsdeathsandmarriages/deaths/bulletins/deathsregisteredinenglandandwalesseriesdr/2017, accessed 13 Oct. 2019.

Pritchard, C., Mayers, A. and Baldwin, D., 2013. Changing patterns of neurological mortality in the 10 major developed countries – 1979–2010. *Public Health, 127*(4), pp.357–68. doi: 10.1016/j.puhe.2012.12.018.

Weinstein, N. D. and Klein, W. M., 1996. Unrealistic optimism: Present and future. *Journal of Social and Clinical Psychology, 15*(1), pp.1–8. doi:10.1521/jscp.1996.15.1.1.

World Health Organization, 22 Mar. 2018. Depression fact sheet. Retrieved from https://www.who.int/news-room/fact-sheets/detail/depression, accessed 16 Feb. 2019.

Zaalberg, A., Nijman, H., Bulten, E., Stroosma, L. and Van Der Staak, C., 2010. Effects of nutritional supplements on aggression, rule-breaking, and psychopathology among young adult prisoners. *Aggressive Behavior: Official Journal of the International Society for Research on Aggression, 36*(2), pp.117–26. doi: 10.1002/ab.20335.

Chapter 2: A Quick Note on Research

Figueroa, T., 2 Nov. 2018. Jury awards $105 million to terminal cancer patient in suit against 'pH Miracle' author. *Los Angeles Times*. Retrieved from https://www.latimes.com/la-me-ln-san-diego-ph-miracle-lawsuit-20181102-story.html, accessed 4 Oct. 2019.

Johnson, S. B., Park, H. S., Gross, C. P. and James, B. Y., 2018. Complementary medicine, refusal of conventional cancer therapy, and survival among patients with curable cancers. *JAMA Oncology*, *4*(10), pp.1375–81. doi:10.1001/jamaoncol.2018.2487.

Chapter 3: Getting to Know the Brain

Cowen, P. J. and Browning, M., 2015. What has serotonin to do with depression? *World Psychiatry*, *14*(2), pp.158–60. doi:10.1002/wps.20229.

Erickson, M. A., Dohi, K. and Banks, W. A., 2012. Neuroinflammation: a common pathway in CNS diseases as mediated at the blood-brain barrier. *N euroimmunomodulation*, *19*(2), pp.121–30. doi:10.1159/000330247.

Hoyle, N. P., Seinkmane, E., Putker, M., Feeney, K. A., Krogager, T. P., Chesham, J. E., Bray, L. K., Thomas, J. M., Dunn, K., Blaikley, J. and O'neill, J. S., 2017. Circadian actin dynamics drive rhythmic fibroblast mobilization during wound healing. *Science Translational Medicine*, *9*(415), p. eaal2774. doi: 10.1126/scitranslmed.aal2774.

Chapter 4: The Major Players

Arsenijevic, Y., Villemure, J. G., Brunet, J. F., Bloch, J. J., Déglon, N., Kostic, C., Zurn, A. and Aebischer, P., 2001. Isolation of multipotent neural precursors residing in the cortex of the adult human brain. *Experimental Neurology*, *170*(1), pp.48–62. doi: 10.1006/exnr.2001.7691.

Autry, A. E. and Monteggia, L. M., 2012. Brain-derived neurotrophic factor and neuropsychiatric disorders. *Pharmacological Reviews*, *64*(2), pp.238–58. doi:10.1124/pr.111.005108.

Etkin, A., Prater, K. E., Schatzberg, A. F., Menon, V. and Greicius, M. D., 2009. Disrupted amygdalar subregion functional connectivity and evidence of a compensatory network in generalized anxiety disorder. *Archives of General Psychiatry, 66*(12), pp.1361–72. doi: 10.1001/ archgenpsychiatry.2009.104.

Frodl, T. S., Koutsouleris, N., Bottlender, R., Born, C., Jäger, M., Scupin, I., Reiser, M., Möller, H. J. and Meisenzahl, E. M., 2008. Depression-related variation in brain morphology over 3 years: effects of stress? *Archives of General Psychiatry, 65*(10), pp.1156–65. doi: 10.1001/archpsyc.65.10.1156.

Katzman, R., Terry, R., DeTeresa, R., Brown, T., Davies, P., Fuld, P., Renbing, X. and Peck, A., 1988. Clinical, pathological, and neurochemical changes in dementia: a subgroup with preserved mental status and numerous neocortical plaques. *Annals of Neurology: Official Journal of the American Neurological Association and the Child Neurology Society, 23*(2), pp.138–44. doi: 10.1002/ana.410230206.

Lam, R. W., Kennedy, S. H., McIntyre, R. S. and Khullar, A., 2014. Cognitive dysfunction in major depressive disorder: effects on psychosocial functioning and implications for treatment. *The Canadian Journal of Psychiatry, 59*(12), pp.649–54. doi:10.1177/070674371405901206.

Maron, E. and Nutt, D., 2017. Biological markers of generalized anxiety disorder. *Dialogues in Clinical Neuroscience, 19*(2), pp.147–58. doi: 10.1176/ appi.focus.16205.

Meng, X. and D'Arcy, C., 2012. Education and dementia in the context of the cognitive reserve hypothesis: a systematic review with meta-analyses and qualitative analyses. *PLOS ONE, 7*(6), p.e38268. doi:10.1371/journal. pone.0038268.

Sharp, E. S. and Gatz, M., 2011. The relationship between education and dementia an updated systematic review. *Alzheimer Disease and Associated Disorders, 25*(4), pp.289–304. doi:10.1097/WAD.0b013e318211c83c.

Yüksel, D., Engelen, J., Schuster, V., Dietsche, B., Konrad, C., Jansen, A., Dannlowski, U., Kircher, T. and Krug, A., 2018. Longitudinal brain volume changes in major depressive disorder. *Journal of Neural Transmission, 125*(10), pp.1433–47. doi: 10.1007/s00702-018-1919-8.

The inflammation hypothesis

Cowen, P. J. and Browning, M., 2015. What has serotonin to do with depression? *World Psychiatry, 14*(2), pp.158–60. doi:10.1002/wps.20229.

Dregan, A., Matcham, F., Harber-Aschan, L., Rayner, L., Brailean, A., Davis, K., Hatch, S., Pariante, C., Armstrong, D., Stewart, R. and Hotopf, M., 2019. Common mental disorders within chronic inflammatory disorders: a primary care database prospective investigation. *Annals of the Rheumatic Diseases*, *78*(5), pp.688–95. doi: 10.1136/annrheumdis-2018-214676.

Grigoleit, J. S., Kullmann, J. S., Wolf, O. T., Hammes, F., Wegner, A., Jablonowski, S., Engler, H., Gizewski, E., Oberbeck, R. and Schedlowski, M., 2011. Dose-dependent effects of endotoxin on neurobehavioral functions in humans. *PLOS ONE*, *6*(12), p.e28330. doi:10.1371/journal.pone.0028330.

Haapakoski, R., Mathieu, J., Ebmeier, K. P., Alenius, H. and Kivimäki, M., 2015. Cumulative meta-analysis of interleukins 6 and 1β, tumour necrosis factor α and C-reactive protein in patients with major depressive disorder. *Brain, Behavior, and Immunity*, *49*, pp.206–15. doi:10.1016/j.bbi.2015.06.001.

Haroon, E., Daguanno, A. W., Woolwine, B. J., Goldsmith, D. R., Baer, W. M., Wommack, E. C., Felger, J. C. and Miller, A. H., 2018. Antidepressant treatment resistance is associated with increased inflammatory markers in patients with major depressive disorder. *Psychoneuroendocrinology*, *95*, pp.43-9. doi:10.1016/j.psyneuen.2018.05.026.

Khairova, R. A., Machado-Vieira, R., Du, J. and Manji, H. K., 2009. A potential role for pro-inflammatory cytokines in regulating synaptic plasticity in major depressive disorder. *International Journal of Neuropsychopharmacology*, *12*(4), pp.561–78. doi: 10.1017/S1461145709009924.

Kotulla, S., Elsenbruch, S., Roderigo, T., Brinkhoff, A., Wegner, A., Engler, H., Schedlowski, M. and Benson, S., 2018. Does human experimental endotoxemia impact negative cognitions related to the self? *Frontiers in Behavioral Neuroscience*, *12*, p.183. doi: 10.3389/fnbeh.2018.00183.

Miller, A. H., Haroon, E., Raison, C. L. and Felger, J. C., 2013. Cytokine targets in the brain: impact on neurotransmitters and neurocircuits. *Depression and Anxiety*, *30*(4), pp.297–306. doi:10.1002/da.22084.

Pariante, C. M., 2017. Why are depressed patients inflamed? A reflection on 20 years of research on depression, glucocorticoid resistance and inflammation. *European Neuropsychopharmacology*, *27*(6), pp.554-9. doi: 10.1016/j.euroneuro.2017.04.001.

Chapter 5: How Stress Affects Brain and Mental Health

Aydemir, O. and Icelli, I., 2013. Burnout: risk factors. In *Burnout for Experts* (pp. 119–43). Springer, Boston, MA.

Calcia, M. A., Bonsall, D. R., Bloomfield, P. S., Selvaraj, S., Barichello, T. and Howes, O. D., 2016. Stress and neuroinflammation: a systematic review of the effects of stress on microglia and the implications for mental illness.
Psychopharmacology, 233(9), pp.1637–50. doi:10.1007/s00213-016-4218-9.

Frick, L. R., Williams, K. and Pittenger, C., 2013. Microglial dysregulation in psychiatric disease. *Clinical and Developmental Immunology, 2013*, 608654. doi:10.1155/2013/608654.

Han, B., Yu, L., Geng, Y., Shen, L., Wang, H., Wang, Y., Wang, J. and Wang, M., 2016. Chronic stress aggravates cognitive impairment and suppresses insulin associated signaling pathway in APP/PS1 mice. *Journal of Alzheimer's Disease, 53*(4), pp.1539–52. doi: 10.3233/JAD-160189.

Katz, M. J., Derby, C. A., Wang, C., Sliwinski, M. J., Ezzati, A., Zimmerman, M. E., Zwerling, J. L. and Lipton, R. B., 2016. Influence of perceived stress on incident amnestic mild cognitive impairment: Results from the Einstein Aging Study. *Alzheimer Disease and Associated Disorders, 30*(2), pp.93–8. doi:10.1097/WAD.0000000000000125.

Kristensen, T. S., Borritz, M., Villadsen, E., & Christensen, K. B. (2005). The Copenhagen Burnout Inventory: A new tool for the assessment of burnout. Work & Stress, 19(3), 192–207.
NHS, 21 May 2018. Medically unexplained symptoms. Retrieved from https://www.nhs.uk/conditions/medically-unexplained-symptoms/, accessed 4 Oct. 2019.

Chapter 6: The Importance of Sleep

Ackerley, R., Badre, G. and Olausson, H., 2015. Positive effects of a weighted blanket on insomnia. *Journal of Sleep Medicine & Disorders, 2*(3), pp.1–7.

Aho, V., Ollila, H. M., Rantanen, V., Kronholm, E., Surakka, I., van Leeuwen, W. M., Lehto, M., Matikainen, S., Ripatti, S., Härmä, M. and Sallinen, M., 2013. Partial sleep restriction activates immune response-related gene expression pathways: experimental and epidemiological studies in humans. *PLOS ONE, 8*(10), p.e77184. doi 10.1371/journal.pone.0077184.

Andrade, C. and Rao, N. S. K., 2010. How antidepressant drugs act: a primer on neuroplasticity as the eventual mediator of antidepressant efficacy. *Indian Journal of Psychiatry, 52*(4), pp.378–86. doi:10.4103/0019-5545.74318.

Bandelow, B. and Michaelis, S., 2015. Epidemiology of anxiety disorders in the 21st century. *Dialogues in Clinical Neuroscience, 17*(3), pp.327–35. PMID: 26487813.

Baron, K. G., Abbott, S., Jao, N., Manalo, N. and Mullen, R., 2017. Orthosomnia: Are some patients taking the quantified self too far? *Journal of Clinical Sleep Medicine, 13*(02), pp.351–4. doi:10.5664/jcsm.6472.

Calvo, J. R., Gonzalez-Yanes, C. and Maldonado, M. D., 2013. The role of melatonin in the cells of the innate immunity: a review. *Journal of Pineal Research, 55*(2), pp.103–20. doi: 10.1111/jpi.12075.

Gosling, J. A., Batterham, P., Ritterband, L., Glozier, N., Thorndike, F., Griffiths, K. M., Mackinnon, A. and Christensen, H. M., 2018. Online insomnia treatment and the reduction of anxiety symptoms as a secondary outcome in a randomised controlled trial: The role of cognitive-behavioural factors. *Australian & New Zealand Journal of Psychiatry, 52*(12), pp.1183–93. doi: 10.1177/0004867418772338.

Martin, P., 2003. The epidemiology of anxiety disorders: a review. *Dialogues in Clinical Neuroscience, 5*(3), pp.281–98. PMID: 22034470.

Pohanka, M., 2013. Impact of melatonin on immunity: a review. *Central European Journal of Medicine, 8*(4), pp.369–76. doi: 10.2478/s11536-013-0177-2.

Sindi, S., Kåreholt, I., Johansson, L., Skoog, J., Sjöberg, L., Wang, H. X., Johansson, B., Fratiglioni, L., Soininen, H., Solomon, A. and Skoog, I., 2018. Sleep disturbances and dementia risk: A multicenter study. *Alzheimer's & Dementia, 14*(10), pp.1235–42. doi: 10.1016/j.jalz.2018.05.012.

Spira, A. P., Chen-Edinboro, L. P., Wu, M. N. and Yaffe, K., 2014. Impact of sleep on the risk of cognitive decline and dementia. *Current Opinion in Psychiatry, 27*(6), pp.478–83. doi:10.1097/YCO.0000000000000106.

Tassi, P. and Muzet, A., 2000. Sleep inertia. *Sleep Medicine Reviews, 4*(4), pp.341–53. doi: 10.1053/smrv.2000.0098.

Vyas, S., Rodrigues, A. J., Silva, J. M., Tronche, F., Almeida, O. F., Sousa, N. and Sotiropoulos, I., 2016. Chronic stress and glucocorticoids: from neuronal plasticity to neurodegeneration. *Neural Plasticity, 2016,* 6391686 doi: 10.1155/2016/6391686.

Xie, L., Kang, H., Xu, Q., Chen, M. J., Liao, Y., Thiyagarajan, M., O'Donnell, J., Christensen, D. J., Nicholson, C., Iliff, J. J. and Takano, T., 2013. Sleep drives metabolite clearance from the adult brain. *Science, 342*(6156), pp.373–77. doi:10.1126/science.1241224.

Yoo, S. S., Gujar, N., Hu, P., Jolesz, F. A. and Walker, M. P., 2007. The human emotional brain without sleep – a prefrontal amygdala disconnect. *Current Biology, 17*(20), pp.R877–8. doi: 10.1016/j.cub.2007.08.007.

Zissermann, L., 1992. The effects of deep pressure on self-stimulating behaviors in a child with autism and other disabilities. *American Journal of Occupational Therapy, 46*(6), pp.547–9. doi:10.5014/ajot.46.6.547.

Chapter 7: Improving Your Brain Health through Nutrition

Adjibade, M., Lemogne, C., Touvier, M., Hercberg, S., Galan, P., Assmann, K. E., Julia, C. and Kesse-Guyot, E., 2019. The inflammatory potential of the diet is directly associated with incident depressive symptoms among French adults. *The Journal of Nutrition, 149*(7), pp. 1198–1207. doi:10.1093/jn/nxz045.

Akbaraly, T. N., Kerleau, C., Wyart, M., Chevallier, N., Ndiaye, L., Shivappa, N., Hébert, J. R. and Kivimäki, M., 2016. Dietary inflammatory index and recurrence of depressive symptoms: results from the Whitehall II Study. *Clinical Psychological Science, 4*(6), pp.1125–34. doi:10.1177/2167702616645777.

Alkasir, R., Li, J., Li, X., Jin, M. and Zhu, B., 2017. Human gut microbiota: the links with dementia development. *Protein & Cell, 8*(2), pp.90–102. doi:10.1007/s13238-016-0338-6.

Ambrosone, C. B., Zirpoli, G. R., Hutson, A. D., McCann, W. E., McCann, S. E., Barlow, W. E., Kelly, K. M., Cannioto, R., Sucheston-Campbell, L. E., Herschman, D. l., Unger, J. M., Moore, H. C. F., Stewart, J. A., Isaacs, C., Hobday, T. J., Salim, M., Hortobagyi, G. N., Gralow, J. R., Budd, G.T & Albain, K. S., 2019. Dietary Supplement Use During Chemotherapy and Survival

Outcomes of Patients With Breast Cancer Enrolled in a Cooperative Group Clinical Trial (SWOG S0221). *Journal of clinical oncology: official journal of the American Society of Clinical Oncology*, JCO1901203. Advance online publication. doi:10.1200/JCO.19.01203

Aranow, C., 2011. Vitamin D and the immune system. *Journal of Investigative Medicine, 59*(6), pp.881–6. doi:10.2310/ JIM.0b013e31821b8755.

Brietzke, E., Cerqueira, R.O., Mansur, R.B. and McIntyre, R.S., 2018. Gluten related illnesses and severe mental disorders: a comprehensive review. *Neuroscience & Biobehavioral Reviews, 84*, pp.368–75. doi:10.1016/ j.neubiorev.2017.08.009.

Brust, J., 2010. Ethanol and cognition: indirect effects, neurotoxicity and neuroprotection: a review. *International Journal of Environmental Research and Public Health, 7*(4), pp.1540–57. doi:10.3390/ijerph7041540.

Cao, D., Kevala, K., Kim, J., Moon, H.-S., Jun, S.B., Lovinger, D. and Kim, H.-Y. (2009), Docosahexaenoic acid promotes hippocampal neuronal development and synaptic function. Journal of Neurochemistry, 111: 510-521. doi:10.1111/j.1471-4159.2009.06335.x

Chassaing, B., Koren, O., Goodrich, J. K., Poole, A. C., Srinivasan, S., Ley, R. E. and Gewirtz, A. T., 2015. Dietary emulsifiers impact the mouse gut microbiota promoting colitis and metabolic syndrome. *Nature, 519*(7541), pp.92–6. doi:10.1038/nature14232. [Published correction appears in *Nature, 536*(7615), p. 238.]

Chassaing, B., Van de Wiele, T., De Bodt, J., Marzorati, M. and Gewirtz, A. T., 2017. Dietary emulsifiers directly alter human microbiota composition and gene expression ex vivo potentiating intestinal inflammation. *Gut, 66*(8), pp.1414–27. doi:10.1136/gutjnl-2016-313099.

Chassaing, B., Vijay-Kumar, M. and Gewirtz, A. T., 2017. How diet can impact gut microbiota to promote or endanger health. *Current Opinion in Gastroenterology, 33*(6), pp.417–21. doi:10.1097/MOG.0000000000000401.

Ciudin, A., Espinosa, A., Simo-Servat, O., Ruiz, A., Alegret, M., Hernandez, C., Boada, M. and Simo, R., 2017. Type 2 diabetes is an independent risk factor for dementia conversion in patients with mild cognitive impairment. *Journal of Diabetes and its Complications, 31*(8), pp.1272–4. doi: 10.1016/j.jdiacomp.2017.04.018.

Collins, M. A., Neafsey, E. J., Mukamal, K. J., Gray, M. O., Parks, D. A., Das, D. K. and Korthuis, R. J., 2009. Alcohol in moderation, cardioprotection, and neuroprotection: epidemiological considerations and mechanistic studies. *Alcoholism: Clinical and Experimental Research, 33*(2), pp.206–19. doi:10.1111/j.1530-0277.2008.00828.x.

Esteban-Cornejo, I., Mota, J., Abreu, S., Pizarro, A. N. and Santos, M. P., 2018. Dietary inflammatory index and academic performance in children. *Public Health Nutrition, 21*(17), pp.3253–7. doi:10.1017/s1368980018001994.

Frith, E., Shivappa, N., Mann, J. R., Hébert, J. R., Wirth, M. D. and Loprinzi, P. D., 2018. Dietary inflammatory index and memory function: population -based national sample of elderly Americans. *British Journal of Nutrition, 119*(5), pp.552–8. doi:10.1017/S0007114517003804.

Groves, N. J., McGrath, J. J. and Burne, T. H., 2014. Vitamin D as a neurosteroid affecting the developing and adult brain. *Annual Review of Nutrition, 34*(1), pp.117–41. doi:10.1146/annurev-nutr-071813-105557.

Gupta, S. and Warner, J., 2008. Alcohol-related dementia: a 21st-century silent epidemic? *The British Journal of Psychiatry, 193*(5), pp.351–3. doi: 10.1192/bjp.bp.108.051425.

Hayden, K. M., Beavers, D. P., Steck, S. E., Hebert, J. R., Tabung, F. K., Shivappa, N., Casanova, R., Manson, J. E., Padula, C. B., Salmoirago-Blotcher, E. and Snetselaar, L. G., 2017. The association between an inflammatory diet and global cognitive function and incident dementia in older women: The Women's Health Initiative Memory Study. *Alzheimer's & Dementia, 13*(11), pp.1187–96. doi:10.1016/j.jalz.2017.04.004.

Hibbeln, J. R., Northstone, K., Evans, J. and Golding, J., 2018. Vegetarian diets and depressive symptoms among men. *Journal of Affective Disorders, 225*, pp.13–17. doi:10.1016/j.jad.2017.07.051.

Jacka, F. N., Pasco, J. A., Mykletun, A., Williams, L. J., Hodge, A. M., O'Reilly, S. L., Nicholson, G. C., Kotowicz, M. A. and Berk, M., 2010. Association of Western and traditional diets with depression and anxiety in women. *American Journal of Psychiatry, 167*(3), pp.305–11. doi:10.1176/ appi.ajp.2009.09060881.

Jackson, J. R., Eaton, W. W., Cascella, N. G., Fasano, A. and Kelly, D. L., 2012. Neurologic and psychiatric manifestations of celiac disease and gluten sensitivity. *Psychiatric Quarterly, 83*(1), pp.91–102. doi:10.1007/s11126-011-9186-y.

Johnston, B. C., Zeraatkar, D., Han, M. A., Vernooij, R. W., Valli, C., El Dib, R., Marshall, C., Stover, P. J., Fairweather-Taitt, S., Wójcik, G. and Bhatia, F., 2019. Unprocessed Red meat and processed meat consumption: Dietary guideline recommendations from the Nutritional Recommendations

(NutriRECS) Consortium. *Annals of Internal Medicine*, [Epub ahead of print 1 Oct. 2019]. doi: 10.7326/M19-1621.

Kharroubi, A. T. and Darwish, H. M., 2015. Diabetes mellitus: The epidemic of the century. *World Journal of Diabetes*, 6(6), pp.850–67. doi:10.4239/wjd.v6.i6.850.

Losurdo, G., Principi, M., Iannone, A., Amoruso, A., Ierardi, E., Di Leo, A. and Barone, M., 2018. Extra-intestinal manifestations of non-celiac gluten sensitivity: An expanding paradigm. *World Journal of Gastroenterology*, 24(14), pp.1521–30. doi:10.3748/wjg.v24.i14.1521.

Luchsinger, J. A., Reitz, C., Patel, B., Tang, M. X., Manly, J. J. and Mayeux, R., 2007. Relation of diabetes to mild cognitive impairment. *Archives of Neurology*, 64(4), pp.570–5. doi:10.1001/archneur.64.4.570.

Michalak, J., Zhang, X. C. and Jacobi, F., 2012. Vegetarian diet and mental disorders: results from a representative community survey. *International Journal of Behavioral Nutrition and Physical Activity*, 9(1), p.67. doi:10.1186/1479-5868-9-67.

Miller, B. J., Whisner, C. M. and Johnston, C. S., 2016. Vitamin D supplementation appears to increase plasma Aβ 40 in vitamin D insufficient older adults: A pilot randomized controlled trial. *Journal of Alzheimer's Disease*, 52(3), pp.843–7. doi:10.3233/jad-150901.

National Health and Nutrition Examination Survey. *Brain, Behavior, and Immunity*, 69, pp.296–303. doi:10.1016/j.bbi.2017.12.003.

NHS, 3 Mar. 2017. Vitamin D. Retrieved from https://www.nhs.uk/conditions/vitamins-and-minerals/vitamin-d/, accessed 4 Oct. 2019.

Ozawa, M., Shipley, M., Kivimaki, M., Singh-Manoux, A. and Brunner, E. J., 2017. Dietary pattern, inflammation and cognitive decline: the Whitehall II prospective cohort study. *Clinical Nutrition*, 36(2), pp.506–12. doi:10.1016/j.clnu.2016.01.013.

Scientific Advisory Committee on Nutrition, 2016. Vitamin D and health. Retrieved from https://assets.publishing.service.gov.uk/government/uploads/system/uploads/attachment_data/file/537616/SACN_Vitamin_D_and_Health_report.pdf, accessed 4 Oct. 2019.

Shivappa, N., Hebert, J. R., Marcos, A., Diaz, L. E., Gomez, S., Nova, E., Michels, N., Arouca, A., González-Gil, E., Frederic, G. and González-Gross, M., 2017. Association between dietary inflammatory index and inflammatory markers in the HELENA study. *Molecular Nutrition & Food Research*, 61(6), p.1600707. doi:10.1002/mnfr.201600707.

Wirth, M. D., Sevoyan, M., Hofseth, L., Shivappa, N., Hurley, T. G. and Hébert, J. R., 2018. The Dietary Inflammatory Index is associated with elevated white blood cell counts in the Public Health England, 17 Mar. 2016. The Eatwell Guide. Retrieved from https://www.gov.uk/government/publications/the-eatwell-guide, accessed 7 Oct. 2019.

Chapter 8: To Fast or Not to Fast

Cheng, C.W., Adams, G.B., Perin, L., Wei, M., Zhou, X., Lam, B.S., Da Sacco, S., Mirisola, M., Quinn, D.I., Dorff, T.B., Kopchick, J.J, Longo VD. Prolonged fasting reduces IGF-1/PKA to promote hematopoietic-stem-cell-based regeneration and reverse immunosuppression. *Cell Stem Cell.* 2014 Jun 5;14(6):810-23. doi: 10.1016/j.stem.2014.04.014. Erratum in: Cell Stem Cell. 2016 Feb 4;18(2):291-2. PMID: 24905167; PMCID: PMC4102383.

Dang, W., 2014. The controversial world of sirtuins. *Drug Discovery Today: Technologies, 12*, pp.e9–e17. doi:10.1016/j.ddtec.2012.08.003.

Fond, G., Macgregor, A., Leboyer, M. and Michalsen, A., 2013. Fasting in mood disorders: neurobiology and effectiveness. A review of the literature. *Psychiatry Research, 209*(3), pp.253–8. doi:10.1016/j.psychres.2012.12.018.

Hornsby, A. K., Redhead, Y. T., Rees, D. J., Ratcliff, M. S., Reichenbach, A., Wells, T., Francis, L., Amstalden, K., Andrews, Z. B. and Davies, J. S., 2016. Short-term calorie restriction enhances adult hippocampal neurogenesis and remote fear memory in a Ghsr-dependent manner. *P sychoneuroendocrinology, 63*, pp.198–207. doi:10.1016/j.psyneuen.2015.09.023.

Jęśko, H., Wencel, P., Strosznajder, R. P. and Strosznajder, J. B., 2017. Sirtuins and their roles in brain aging and neurodegenerative disorders. *Neurochemical Research, 42*(3), pp.876–90. doi:10.1007/s11064-016-2110-y.

Kent, B. A., Beynon, A. L., Hornsby, A. K., Bekinschtein, P., Bussey, T. J., Davies, J. S. and Saksida, L. M., 2015. The orexigenic hormone acyl-ghrelin increases adult hippocampal neurogenesis and enhances pattern separation. *Psychoneuroendocrinology, 51*, pp.431–9. doi:10.1016/j.psyneuen.2014.10.015.

Lutz, M. I., Milenkovic, I., Regelsberger, G. and Kovacs, G. G., 2014. Distinct patterns of sirtuin expression during progression of Alzheimer's disease. *Neuromolecular Medicine, 16*(2), pp.405–14. doi:10.1007/s12017-014-8288-8.

Martin, B., Mattson, M. P. and Maudsley, S., 2006. Caloric restriction and intermittent fasting: Two potential diets for successful brain aging. *Ageing Research Reviews, 5*(3), pp.332–53. doi:10.1016/j.arr.2006.04.002.

Siegel, J. M., 2004. Hypocretin (OREXIN): Role in normal behavior and neuropathology. *Annual Review of Psychology, 55,* pp.125–48. doi:10.1146/annurev.psych.55.090902.141.

Spencer, S. J., Xu, L., Clarke, M. A., Lemus, M., Reichenbach, A., Geenen, B., Kozicz, T. and Andrews, Z. B., 2012. Ghrelin regulates the hypothalamic-pituitary-adrenal axis and restricts anxiety after acute stress. *Biological Psychiatry, 72*(6), pp.457–65. doi:10.1016/j.biopsych.2012.03.010.

Walsh, J. J., Edgett, B. A., Tschakovsky, M. E. and Gurd, B. J., 2014. Fasting and exercise differentially regulate BDNF mRNA expression in human skeletal muscle. *Applied Physiology, Nutrition, and Metabolism, 40*(1), pp.96–8. doi:10.1139/apnm-2014-0290.

Witte, A. V., Fobker, M., Gellner, R., Knecht, S. and Flöel, A., 2009. Caloric restriction improves memory in elderly humans. *Proceedings of the National Academy of Sciences, 106*(4), pp.1255–60. doi:10.1073/pnas.0808587106.

Zhang, Y., Liu, C., Zhao, Y., Zhang, X., Li, B. and Cui, R., 2015. The effects of calorie restriction in depression and potential mechanisms. *Current Neuropharmacology, 13*(4), pp.536–42. doi:10.2174/1570159X13666150326003852.

Chapter 9: How Physical Activity Protects the Brain

ABC News, 31 Jul. 2018. NFL concussion settlement payouts reach $US500 million after two years, already more than estimates for a decade. Retrieved from https://www.abc.net.au/news/2018-07-31/nfl-concussion-claims-outstrip-predictions-decade-in-two-years/10056496, accessed 7 Oct. 2019.

Audible [no date]. The Beautiful Brain: Omalu, B. Interview with Hana Walker-Brown [podcast]. Retrieved from https://www.audible.co.uk/pd/The-Beautiful-Brain, accessed 7 Oct. 2019.

Berrueta, L., Muskaj, I., Olenich, S., Butler, T., Badger, G. J., Colas, R. A., Spite, M., Serhan, C. N. and Langevin, H. M., 2016. Stretching impacts inflammation resolution in connective tissue. *Journal of Cellular Physiology*, *231*(7), pp.1621–7. doi:10.1002/jcp.25263.

Bolandzadeh, N., Tam, R., Handy, T. C., Nagamatsu, L. S., Hsu, C. L., Davis, J. C., Dao, E., Beattie, B. L. and Liu-Ambrose, T., 2015. Resistance training and white matter lesion progression in older women: Exploratory analysis of a 12-month randomized controlled trial. *Journal of the American Geriatrics Society*, *63*(10), pp.2052–60. doi:10.1111/jgs.13644.

Boston University Center for the Study of Traumatic Encephalopathy, 17 October 2014. Image of chronic traumatic encephalopathy. Source: www-tc.pbs.org/wgbh/pages/frontline/art/progs/concussions-cte/h.png, accessed 9 Jan. 2020.

Choi, K. W., Zheutlin, A. B., Karlson, R. A., Wang, M. J., Dunn, E. C., Stein, M. B., Karlson, E.W. & Smoller, J. W., 2019. Physical activity offsets genetic risk for incident depression assessed via electronic health records in a biobank cohort study. *Depression and Anxiety*. doi.org/10.1002/da.22967

Fernandes, J., Arida, R. M. and Gomez-Pinilla, F., 2017. Physical exercise as an epigenetic modulator of brain plasticity and cognition. *Neuroscience & Biobehavioral Reviews*, *80*, pp.443–56. doi:10.1016/j.neubiorev.2017.06.012.

Ferris, L. T., Williams, J. S. and Shen, C. L., 2007. The effect of acute exercise on serum brain-derived neurotrophic factor levels and cognitive function. *Medicine and Science in Sports and Exercise*, *39*(4), pp.728–34. doi:10.1249/mss.0b013e31802f04c7.
Hamer, M., Endrighi, R. and Poole, L., 2012. Physical activity, stress reduction, and mood: Insight into immunological mechanisms. In Yan, Q. (eds). *Psychoneuroimmunology: Methods in molecular biology (methods and protocols)*, *934*, pp. 89–102. Humana Press, Totowa, NJ. doi:10.1007/978-1-62703-071-7_5.

Hamer, M., Stamatakis, E. and Steptoe, A., 2009. Dose-response relationship between physical activity and mental health: The Scottish Health Survey. *British Journal of Sports Medicine*, *43*(14), pp.1111–14. doi: 10.1136/bjsm.2008.046243.

Hoskins, A. and Hooker, R. S., 2015. Sudden impact: Concussion incidence in female roller derby athletes. *Journal of the American Academy of Physician Assistants*, *28*(11), p.1. doi:10.1097/01.jaa.0000471292.02985.6a.

Jeon, Y. K. and Ha, C. H., 2017. The effect of exercise intensity on brain derived neurotrophic factor and memory in adolescents. *Environmental Health and Preventive Medicine*, 22(1), p.27. doi:10.1186/s12199-017-0643-6.

Kempton, M. J., Ettinger, U., Foster, R., Williams, S. C., Calvert, G. A., Hampshire, A., Zelaya, F. O., O'Gorman, R. L., McMorris, T., Owen, A. M. and Smith, M. S., 2011. Dehydration affects brain structure and function in healthy adolescents. *Human Brain Mapping*, 32(1), pp.71–9. doi:10.1002/hbm.20999.

Lakhan, S. E. and Kirchgessner, A., 2012. Chronic traumatic encephalopathy: the dangers of getting "dinged". *SpringerPlus*, 1(1), p.2. doi: 10.1186/2193-1801-1-2.

Mandolesi, L., Polverino, A., Montuori, S., Foti, F., Ferraioli, G., Sorrentino, P. and Sorrentino, G., 2018. Effects of physical exercise on cognitive functioning and wellbeing: Biological and psychological benefits. *Frontiers in Psychology*, 9, p.509. doi:10.3389/fpsyg.2018.00509.

Maroon, J. C., LePere, D. B., Blaylock, R. L. and Bost, J. W., 2012. Postconcussion syndrome: A review of pathophysiology and potential nonpharmacological approaches to treatment. *The Physician and Sportsmedicine*, 40(4), pp.73–87. doi:10.3810/psm.2012.11.1990.

Mez, J., Daneshvar, D. H., Kiernan, P. T., Abdolmohammadi, B., Alvarez, V. E., Huber, B. R., Alosco, M. L., Solomon, T. M., Nowinski, C. J., McHale, L. and Cormier, K. A., 2017. Clinicopathological evaluation of chronic traumatic encephalopathy in players of American football. *JAMA*, 318(4), pp.360–70. doi:10.1001/jama.2017.8334.

NFL Concussion Settlement [no date]. Retrieved from https://www.nflconcussionsettlement.com/Home.aspx, accessed 7 Oct. 2019.

Omalu, B. I., Fitzsimmons, R. P., Hammers, J. and Bailes, J., 2010. Chronic traumatic encephalopathy in a professional American wrestler. *Journal of Forensic Nursing*, 6(3), pp.130–6. doi:10.1111/j.1939-3938.2010.01078.x.

Public Broadcasting Service [no date]. League of denial: The NFL's concussion crisis. Retrieved from https://www.pbs.org/wgbh/pages/frontline/oral-history/league-of-denial/, accessed 7 Oct. 2019.

Stern, R. A., Riley, D. O., Daneshvar, D. H., Nowinski, C. J., Cantu, R. C. and McKee, A. C., 2011. Long-term consequences of repetitive brain trauma: chronic traumatic encephalopathy. *PM&R*, 3(10), pp.S460–7. doi:10.1016/j.pmrj.2011.08.008.

Tyndall, A. V., Clark, C. M., Anderson, T. J., Hogan, D. B., Hill, M. D., Longman, R. S. and Poulin, M. J., 2018. Protective effects of exercise on cognition and brain health in older adults. *Exercise and Sport Sciences Reviews*, 46(4), pp.215–23. doi:10.1249/jes.0000000000000161.

Van Cutsem, J., Pattyn, N., Vissenaeken, D., Dhondt, G., De Pauw, K., Tonoli, C., Meeusen, R. and Roelands, B., 2015. The influence of a mild thermal challenge and severe hypoxia on exercise performance and serum BDNF. *European Journal of Applied Physiology*, 115(10), pp.2135–48. doi:10.1007/s00421-015-3193-x.

World Health Organization, 2010. Global Recommendations on Physical Activity for Health. WHO Press.

Why yoga works

Schumann, D., Langhorst, J., Dobos, G. and Cramer, H., 2018. Randomised clinical trial: Yoga vs a low-FODMAP diet in patients with irritable bowel syndrome. *Alimentary Pharmacology & Therapeutics*, 47(2), pp.203–11. doi:10.1111/apt.14400.

Chapter 10: Using the Breath

Boksa, P., 2017. Smoking, psychiatric illness and the brain. *Journal of Psychiatry & Neuroscience*, 42(3), pp.147–9. doi:10.1503/jpn.170060.
Bonaz, B., Sinniger, V. and Pellissier, S., 2016. Anti-inflammatory properties of the vagus nerve: Potential therapeutic implications of vagus nerve stimulation. *The Journal of Physiology*, 594(20), pp.5781–90. doi:10.1113/JP271539.

Borovikova, L. V., Ivanova, S., Zhang, M., Yang, H., Botchkina, G. I., Watkins, L. R., Wang, H., Abumrad, N., Eaton, J. W. and Tracey, K. J., 2000. Vagus nerve stimulation attenuates the systemic inflammatory response to endotoxin. *Nature*, 405(6785), pp.458–62. doi:10.1038/35013070.

Brown, R. P. and Gerbarg, P. L., 2005. Sudarshan Kriya yogic breathing in the treatment of stress, anxiety, and depression: Part I – neurophysiologic model. *The Journal of Alternative and Complementary Medicine*, 11(1), pp.189–201. doi:10.1089/acm.2005.11.189

Brown, R. P., Gerbarg, P. L. and Muench, F., 2013. Breathing practices for treatment of psychiatric and stress-related medical conditions. *Psychiatric Clinics of North America, 36*(1), pp.121–40. doi:10.1016/j.psc.2013.01.001.

Chen, H., Kwong, J. C., Copes, R., Tu, K., Villeneuve, P. J., Van Donkelaar, A., Hystad, P., Martin, R. V., Murray, B. J., Jessiman, B. and Wilton, A. S., 2017. Living near major roads and the incidence of dementia, Parkinson's disease, and multiple sclerosis: A population-based cohort study. *The Lancet, 389*(10070), pp.718–26. doi:10.1016/s0140-6736(16)32399-6.

Durazzo, T. C., Meyerhoff, D. J. and Nixon, S. J., 2010. Chronic cigarette smoking: Implications for neurocognition and brain neurobiology. *International Journal of Environmental Research and Public Health, 7*(10), pp.3760–91. doi:10.3390/ijerph7103760.

Kalyani, B. G., Venkatasubramanian, G., Arasappa, R., Rao, N. P., Kalmady, S. V., Behere, R. V., Rao, H., Vasudev, M. K. and Gangadhar, B. N., 2011. Neurohemodynamic correlates of 'OM' chanting: A pilot functional magnetic resonance imaging study. *International Journal of Yoga, 4*(1), pp.3–6. doi:10.4103/0973-6131.78171.

Kang, J., Scholp, A. and Jiang, J. J., 2018. A review of the physiological effects and mechanisms of singing. *Journal of Voice, 32*(4), pp.390–5. doi:10.1016/j.jvoice.2017.07.008.

Karama, S., Ducharme, S., Corley, J., Chouinard-Decorte, F., Starr, J. M., Wardlaw, J. M., Bastin, M. E. and Deary, I. J., 2015. Cigarette smoking and thinning of the brain's cortex. *Molecular Psychiatry, 20*(6), pp.778–85. doi:10.1038/mp.2014.187.

Koopman, F. A., Musters, A., Backer, M. J., Gerlag, D., Miljko, S., Grazio, S., Sokolovic, S., Levine, Y. A., Chernoff, D., de Vries, N. and Tak, P. P., 2018. SAT0240 Vagus nerve stimulation in patients with rheumatoid arthritis: Two-year safety and efficacy. *Annals of the Rheumatic Diseases, 77*, pp.981–2. doi: 10.1136/annrheumdis-2018-eular.1802.

National Institute for Health and Care Excellence, Dec. 2009. Vagus nerve stimulation for treatment-resistant depression. Retrieved from https://www.nice.org.uk/guidance/ipg330/chapter/1-Guidance, accessed 7 Oct. 2019.

Sharma, A., Barrett, M. S., Cucchiara, A. J., Gooneratne, N. S. and Thase, M. E., 2017. A breathing-based meditation intervention for patients with major depressive disorder following inadequate response to antidepressants: A randomized pilot study. *The Journal of Clinical Psychiatry, 78*(1), pp.e59–63. doi:10.4088/JCP.16m10819.

Valenza, M. C., Valenza-Peña, G., Torres-Sánchez, I., González-Jiménez, E., Conde-Valero, A. and Valenza-Demet, G., 2014. Effectiveness of controlled breathing techniques on anxiety and depression in hospitalized patients with COPD: A randomized clinical trial. *Respiratory Care, 59*(2), pp.209–15. doi:10.4187/respcare.02565.

Zelano, C., Jiang, H., Zhou, G., Arora, N., Schuele, S., Rosenow, J. and Gottfried, J. A., 2016. Nasal respiration entrains human limbic oscillations and modulates cognitive function. *Journal of Neuroscience, 36*(49), pp.12448–67. doi:10.1523/jneurosci.2586-16.2016.

Zhang, X., Chen, X. and Zhang, X., 2018. The impact of exposure to air pollution on cognitive performance. *Proceedings of the National Academy of Sciences, 115*(37), pp.9193–7. doi:10.1073/pnas.1809474115.

Chapter 11: Understanding Emotions

Chapman, B. P., Fiscella, K., Kawachi, I., Duberstein, P. and Muennig, P., 2013. Emotion suppression and mortality risk over a 12-year follow-up. *Journal of Psychosomatic Research, 75*(4), pp.381–5. doi:10.1016/j.jpsychores.2013.07.014.

Côté, M., Gagnon-Girouard, M. P., Sabourin, S. and Bégin, C., 2018. Emotion suppression and food intake in the context of a couple discussion: A dyadic analysis. *Appetite, 120*, pp.109–14. doi:10.1016/j.appet.2017.08.029.

Ferrer, R. A., Green, P. A., Oh, A. Y., Hennessy, E. and Dwyer, L. A., 2017. Emotion suppression, emotional eating, and eating behavior among parent–adolescent dyads. *Emotion, 17*(7), pp.1052–65. doi:10.1037/emo0000295.

Freund, V. and Frossard, N., 2004. Expression of nerve growth factor in the airways and its possible role in asthma. *Progress in Brain Research, 146*, pp.335–46. doi:10.1016/s0079-6123(03)46021-4.

Gračanin, A., Vingerhoets, A. J., Kardum, I., Zupčić, M., Šantek, M. and Šimić, M., 2015. Why crying does and sometimes does not seem to alleviate mood: A quasi-experimental study. *Motivation and Emotion, 39*(6), pp.953–60. doi:10.1007/s11031-015-9507-9.

Hasson, O., 2009. Emotional tears as biological signals. *Evolutionary Psychology, 7*(3), p.147470490900700302. doi:10.1177/147470490900700302.

Kaplow, J. B., Gipson, P. Y., Horwitz, A. G., Burch, B. N. and King, C. A., 2014. Emotional suppression mediates the relation between adverse life events and adolescent suicide: Implications for prevention. *Prevention Science*, 15(2), pp.177–85. doi:10.1007/s11121-013-0367-9.

Roberts, N. A., Levenson, R. W. and Gross, J. J., 2008. Cardiovascular costs of emotion suppression cross ethnic lines. *International Journal of Psychophysiology*, 70(1), pp.82–7. doi:10.1016/j.ijpsycho.2008.06.003.

Sznycer, D., Xygalatas, D., Agey, E., Alami, S., An, X. F., Ananyeva, K. I., Atkinson, Q. D., Broitman, B. R., Conte, T. J., Flores, C. and Fukushima, S., 2018. Cross-cultural invariances in the architecture of shame. *Proceedings of the National Academy of Sciences*, 115(39), pp.9702–7. doi:10.1073/pnas.1805016115.

Tull, M. T., Jakupcak, M. and Roemer, L., 2010. Emotion suppression: A preliminary experimental investigation of its immediate effects and role in subsequent reactivity to novel stimuli. *Cognitive Behaviour Therapy*, 39(2), pp.114–25. doi:10.1080/16506070903280491.

Vingerhoets, A. J. and Bylsma, L. M., 2016. The riddle of human emotional crying: A challenge for emotion researchers. *Emotion Review*, 8(3), pp.207–17. doi:10.1177/1754073915586226.

Chapter 12: Building Psychological Resilience

Alghasham, A. and Rasheed, N., 2014. Stress-mediated modulations in dopaminergic system and their subsequent impact on behavioral and oxidative alterations: An update. *Pharmaceutical Biology*, 52(3), pp.368–77. doi: 10.3109/13880209.2013.837492.

Amati, V., Meggiolaro, S., Rivellini, G. and Zaccarin, S., 2018. Social relations and life satisfaction: The role of friends. *Genus*, 74(1), p.7. doi:10.1186/s41118-018-0032-z.

Germer, C. K. and Neff, K. D., 2013. Self-compassion in clinical practice. *Journal of Clinical Psychology*, 69(8), pp.856–67. doi:10.1002/jclp.22021.

Hill, P. L. and Turiano, N. A., 2014. Purpose in life as a predictor of mortality across adulthood. *Psychological Science*, 25(7), pp.1482–6. doi:10.1177/0956797614531799.

Hill, P. L., Turiano, N. A., Mroczek, D. K. and Burrow, A. L., 2016. The value of a purposeful life: Sense of purpose predicts greater income and net worth. *Journal of Research in Personality, 65*, pp.38–42. doi:10.1016/j.jrp.2016.07.003.

Ho, C. Y., 2016. Better health with more friends: The role of social capital in producing health. *Health Economics, 25*(1), pp.91–100. doi:10.1002/hec.3131.

Leach, J., 2018. 'Give-up-itis' revisited: Neuropathology of extremis. *Medical Hypotheses, 120*, pp.14–21. doi:10.1016/j.mehy.2018.08.009.

Musich, S., Wang, S. S., Kraemer, S., Hawkins, K. and Wicker, E., 2018. Purpose in life and positive health outcomes among older adults. *Population Health Management, 21*(2), pp.139–47. doi:10.1089/pop.2017.0063.

Ozbay, F., Johnson, D. C., Dimoulas, E., Morgan III, C. A., Charney, D. and Southwick, S., 2007. Social support and resilience to stress: From neurobiology to clinical practice. *Psychiatry (Edgmont), 4*(5), pp.35–40. PMID: 20806028.

Silverman, M. N. and Deuster, P. A., 2014. Biological mechanisms underlying the role of physical fitness in health and resilience. *Interface Focus, 4*(5), p.20140040. doi:10.1098/rsfs.2014.0040.

Southwick, S. and Charney, D., 2012, *Resilience: The Secret To Mastering Life's Greatest Challenges.* Cambridge: Cambridge University Press.

Southwick, S. M. and Charney, D. S., 2012. The science of resilience: Implications for the prevention and treatment of depression. *Science, 338*(6103), pp.79–82. doi:10.1126/science.1222942.

Sutin, A. R., Stephan, Y., Luchetti, M. and Terracciano, A., 2018. Loneliness and risk of dementia. *The Journals of Gerontology: Series B.* doi:10.1093/geronb/gby112.

Tomioka, K., Kurumatani, N. and Hosoi, H., 2016. Relationship of having hobbies and a purpose in life with mortality, activities of daily living, and instrumental activities of daily living among community-dwelling elderly adults. *Journal of Epidemiology, 26*(7), pp.361–70. doi:10.2188/jea.JE20150153.

Van Harmelen, A. L., Kievit, R. A., Ioannidis, K., Neufeld, S., Jones, P. B., Bullmore, E., Dolan, R., Fonagy, P., Goodyer, I. and NSPN Consortium, 2017. Adolescent friendships predict later resilient functioning across psychosocial domains in a healthy community cohort. *Psychological Medicine, 47*(13), pp.2312–22. doi:10.1017/s0033291717000836.

Wallace, L. E., Anthony, R., End, C. M. and Way, B. M., 2019. Does religion stave off the grave? Religious affiliation in one's obituary and longevity. *Social Psychological and Personality Science, 10*(5), pp.662–70. doi:10.1177/1948550618779820.

Chapter 13: Other Lifestyle Factors That Impact Brain Health

Heat

Hanusch, K. U., Janssen, C. H., Billheimer, D., Jenkins, I., Spurgeon, E., Lowry, C. A. and Raison, C. L., 2013. Whole-body hyperthermia for the treatment of major depression: Associations with thermoregulatory cooling. *American Journal of Psychiatry, 170*(7), pp.802–4. doi:10.1176/appi.ajp.2013.12111395.

Hussain, J. and Cohen, M., 2018. Clinical effects of regular dry sauna bathing: A systematic review. *Evidence-Based Complementary and Alternative Medicine, 2018*, 1857413. doi:10.1155/2018/1857413.

IJzerman, H. and Semin, G. R., 2009. The thermometer of social relations: Mapping social proximity on temperature. *Psychological Science, 20*(10), pp.1214–20. doi:10.1111/j.1467-9280.2009.02434.x.

Janssen, C. W., Lowry, C. A., Mehl, M. R., Allen, J. J., Kelly, K. L., Gartner, D. E., Medrano, A., Begay, T. K., Rentscher, K., White, J. J. and Fridman, A., 2016. Whole-body hyperthermia for the treatment of major depressive disorder: A randomized clinical trial. *JAMA Psychiatry, 73*(8), pp.789–95. doi:10.1001/jamapsychiatry.2016.1031.

Kunutsor, S. K., Laukkanen, T. and Laukkanen, J. A., 2018. Longitudinal associations of sauna bathing with inflammation and oxidative stress: The KIHD prospective cohort study. *Annals of Medicine, 50*(5), pp.437–42. doi:10.1080/07853890.2018.1489143.

Laukkanen, J. A. and Laukkanen, T., 2018. Sauna bathing and systemic inflammation. *European Journal of Epidemiology, 33*(3), pp.351–3. doi:10.1007/s10654-017-0335-y.

Laukkanen, T., Kunutsor, S., Kauhanen, J. and Laukkanen, J. A., 2016. Sauna bathing is inversely associated with dementia and Alzheimer's disease in middle-aged Finnish men. *Age and Ageing, 46*(2), pp.245–9. doi: 10.1093/ageing/afw212.

Laukkanen, T., Laukkanen, J. A. and Kunutsor, S. K., 2018. Sauna bathing and risk of psychotic disorders: A prospective cohort study. *Medical Principles and Practice, 27*(6), pp.562–9. doi: 10.1159/000493392.

Leak, R. K., 2014. Heat shock proteins in neurodegenerative disorders and aging. *Journal of Cell Communication and Signaling, 8*(4), pp.293–310. doi:10.1007/s12079-014-0243-9.

Masuda, A., Nakazato, M., Kihara, T., Minagoe, S. and Tei, C., 2005. Repeated thermal therapy diminishes appetite loss and subjective complaints in mildly depressed patients. *Psychosomatic Medicine, 67*(4), pp.643–7. doi:10.1097/01.psy.0000171812.67767.8f.

Raison, C. L., Hale, M. W., Williams, L., Wager, T. D. and Lowry, C. A., 2015. Somatic influences on subjective well-being and affective disorders: The convergence of thermosensory and central serotonergic systems. *Frontiers in Psychology, 5*, p.1580. doi:10.3389/fpsyg.2014.01580.

Robins, H. I., Kalin, N. H., Shelton, S. E., Martin, P. A., Shecterle, L. M., Barksdale, C. M., Neville, A. J. and Marshall, J., 1987. Rise in plasma beta-endorphin, ACTH, and cortisol in cancer patients undergoing whole body hyperthermia. *Hormone and Metabolic Research, 19*(09), pp.441–3. doi:10.1055/s-2007-1011847.

Williams, L. E. and Bargh, J. A., 2008. Experiencing physical warmth promotes interpersonal warmth. *Science, 322*(5901), pp.606–7. doi:10.1126/science.1162548.

Paying attention

Hölzel, B. K., Carmody, J., Vangel, M., Congleton, C., Yerramsetti, S. M., Gard, T. and Lazar, S. W., 2011. Mindfulness practice leads to increases in regional brain gray matter density. *Psychiatry Research: Neuroimaging, 191*(1), pp.36–43. doi:10.1016/j.pscychresns.2010.08.006.

Lazar, S. W., Kerr, C. E., Wasserman, R. H., Gray, J. R., Greve, D. N., Treadway, M. T., McGarvey, M., Quinn, B. T., Dusek, J. A., Benson, H. and Rauch, S. L., 2005. Meditation experience is associated with increased cortical thickness. *Neuroreport, 16*(17), pp.1893–7. doi:10.1097/01.wnr.0000186598.66243.19.

Maron, E. and Nutt, D., 2017. Biological markers of generalized anxiety disorder. *Dialogues in Clinical Neuroscience, 19*(2), pp.147–58. doi: 10.1176/appi.focus.16205.

Xu, W., Tan, L., Wang, H. F., Tan, M. S., Tan, L., Li, J. Q., Zhao, Q. F. and Yu, J. T., 2016. Education and risk of dementia: Dose-response meta-analysis of prospective cohort studies. *Molecular Neurobiology, 53*(5), pp.3113–23. doi:10.1007/s12035-015-9211-5.

Dental health

Aeberli, I., Gerber, P. A., Hochuli, M., Kohler, S., Haile, S. R., Gouni-Berthold, I., Berthold, H. K., Spinas, G. A. and Berneis, K., 2011. Low to moderate sugar-sweetened beverage consumption impairs glucose and lipid metabolism and promotes inflammation in healthy young men: A randomized controlled trial. *The American Journal of Clinical Nutrition, 94*(2), pp.479–85. doi:10.3945/ajcn.111.013540.

Barnes, J. N. and Joyner, M. J., 2012. Sugar highs and lows: the impact of diet on cognitive function. *The Journal of Physiology, 590*(12), p.2831. doi:10.1113/jphysiol.2012.234328.

British Dental Association [no date]. Myth busters on brushing your teeth. Retrieved from https://bda.org/about-the-bda/campaigns/oralhealth/Pages/brushing-myth-busters.aspx, accessed 7 Oct. 2019.

Chen, C. K., Wu, Y. T. and Chang, Y. C., 2017. Association between chronic periodontitis and the risk of Alzheimer's disease: A retrospective, population-based, matched-cohort study. *Alzheimer's Research & Therapy, 9*(1), p.56. doi:10.1186/s13195-017-0282-6.

Chiang, C. H., Wu, M. P., Ho, C. H., Weng, S. F., Huang, C. C., Hsieh, W. T., Hsu, Y. W. and Chen, P. J., 2015. Lower urinary tract symptoms are associated with increased risk of dementia among the elderly: A nationwide study. *BioMed Research International, 2015*, 187819. doi:10.1155/2015/187819.

Dominy, S. S., Lynch, C., Ermini, F., Benedyk, M., Marczyk, A., Konradi, A., Nguyen, M., Haditsch, U., Raha, D., Griffin, C. and Holsinger, L. J., 2019. Porphyromonas gingivalis in Alzheimer's disease brains: Evidence for disease causation and treatment with small-molecule inhibitors. *Science Advances, 5*(1), p.eaau3333. doi:10.1126/sciadv.aau3333.

Freeman, C. R., Zehra, A., Ramirez, V., Wiers, C. E., Volkow, N. D. and Wang, G. J., 2018. Impact of sugar on the body, brain, and behavior. *Frontiers in Bioscience)*, *23*, pp.2255–66. PMID: 29772560.

Gosztyla, M. L., Brothers, H. M. and Robinson, S. R., 2018. Alzheimer's amyloid-β is an antimicrobial peptide: A review of the evidence. *Journal of Alzheimer's Disease, 62*(4), pp.1495–506. doi:10.3233/jad-171133.

Ilievski, V., Zuchowska, P. K., Green, S. J., Toth, P. T., Ragozzino, M. E., Le, K., Aljewari, H. W., O'Brien-Simpson, N. M., Reynolds, E. C. and Watanabe, K., 2018. Chronic oral application of a periodontal pathogen results in brain inflammation, neurodegeneration and amyloid beta production in wild type mice. *PLOS ONE*, *13*(10), p.e0204941. doi:10.1371/journal. pone.0204941.

Ishida, N., Ishihara, Y., Ishida, K., Tada, H., Funaki-Kato, Y., Hagiwara, M., Ferdous, T., Abdullah, M., Mitani, A., Michikawa, M. and Matsushita, K., 2017. Periodontitis induced by bacterial infection exacerbates features of Alzheimer's disease in transgenic mice. *NPJ Aging and Mechanisms of Disease*, *3*(1), p.15. doi:10.1038/s41514-017-0015-x.

Kumar, D. K. V., Choi, S. H., Washicosky, K. J., Eimer, W. A., Tucker, S., Ghofrani, J., Lefkowitz, A., McColl, G., Goldstein, L. E., Tanzi, R. E. and Moir, R. D., 2016. Amyloid-β peptide protects against microbial infection in mouse and worm models of Alzheimer's disease. *Science Translational Medicine*, *8*(340), pp.340ra72. doi:10.1126/scitranslmed.aaf1059.

NHS, 2 Apr. 2019. Tooth decay. Retrieved from https://www.nhs.uk/conditions/tooth-decay/, accessed 7 Oct. 2019.

Omenn, G. S., Goodman, G. E., Thornquist, M. D., Balmes, J., Cullen, M. R., Glass, A., Keogh, J. P., Meyskens Jr, F. L., Valanis, B., Williams Jr, J. H. and Barnhart, S., 1996. Risk factors for lung cancer and for intervention effects in CARET, the Beta-Carotene and Retinol Efficacy Trial. *JNCI: Journal of the National Cancer Institute*, *88*(21), pp.1550–59. doi.org/10.1093/jnci/88.21.1550.

Pase, M. P., Himali, J. J., Jacques, P. F., DeCarli, C., Satizabal, C. L., Aparicio, H., Vasan, R. S., Beiser, A. S. and Seshadri, S., 2017. Sugary beverage intake and preclinical Alzheimer's disease in the community. *Alzheimer's & Dementia*, *13*(9), pp.955–64. doi:10.1016/j.jalz.2017.01.024.

Poole, S., Singhrao, S. K., Chukkapalli, S., Rivera, M., Velsko, I., Kesavalu, L. and Crean, S., 2015. Active invasion of Porphyromonas gingivalis and infection-induced complement activation in ApoE-/- mice brains. *Journal of Alzheimer's Disease*, *43*(1), pp.67–80. doi:10.3233/jad-140315.

Public Health England, Mar. 2018. National diet and nutrition survey. Retrieved from https://assets.publishing.service.gov.uk/government/uploads/system/uploads/attachment_data/file/699241/NDNS_results_years_7_and_8.pdf, accessed 7 Oct. 2019.

Singhrao, S. K., Harding, A., Simmons, T., Robinson, S., Kesavalu, L. and Crean, S., 2014. Oral inflammation, tooth loss, risk factors, and association with progression of Alzheimer's disease. *Journal of Alzheimer's Disease, 42*(3), pp.723–37. doi:10.3233/jad-140387.

Chapter 14: How Social Media and Technology Affect the Brain

Apter, T., 2019. Disrupting the feed. Teenage girls' use of social media: an intervention to improve social media health. Retrieved from https://zzjyl3l-hxs3eyvm92cs1kx1a-wpengine.netdna-ssl.com/wp-content/uploads/2019/10/Research-Results-July-2019.pdf, accessed 13 Oct. 2019.

Dwyer, R. J., Kushlev, K. and Dunn, E. W., 2018. Smartphone use undermines enjoyment of face-to-face social interactions. *Journal of Experimental Social Psychology, 78*, pp.233–9. doi: 10.1016/j.jesp.2017.10.007.

Kushlev, K., Dwyer, R. and Dunn, E. W., 2019. The social price of constant connectivity: Smartphones impose subtle costs on well-being. *Current Directions in Psychological Science*, p.0963721419847200. doi:10.1177/0963721419847200.

Mueller, P. A. and Oppenheimer, D. M., 2014. The pen is mightier than the keyboard: Advantages of longhand over laptop note taking. *Psychological Science, 25*(6), pp.1159–68. doi:10.1177/0956797614524581.

Ozimek, P. and Bierhoff, H. W., 2019. All my online-friends are better than me – three studies about ability-based comparative social media use, self-esteem, and depressive tendencies. *Behaviour & Information Technology*, pp.1-14. doi:10.1080/0144929x.2019.1642385.

Park, S. Y. and Baek, Y. M., 2018. Two faces of social comparison on Facebook: The interplay between social comparison orientation, emotions, and psychological well-being. *Computers in Human Behavior, 79*, pp.83–93. doi:10.1016/j.chb.2017.10.028.

Parker, S., 11 Nov. 2017. Facebook exploits human vulnerability (we are dopamine addicts) [video], YouTube. Retrieved from https://www.youtube.com/watch?v=R7jar4KgKxs, accessed 7 Oct. 2019.

Ward, A. F., Duke, K., Gneezy, A. and Bos, M. W., 2017. Brain drain: The mere presence of one's own smartphone reduces available cognitive capacity. *Journal of the Association for Consumer Research*, 2(2), pp.140–54. doi:10.1086/691462.

The health risks of fake news and how critical thinking can help

Graham, P., Mar. 2008. How to disagree. Retrieved from http://www. paulgraham.com/disagree.html, accessed 7 Oct. 2019.

Walton, G., Wilkinson, A., Turner, M., Pointon, M. and Barker, J., 2018. Measuring the psychophysiology of information literacy. In *The Sixth European Conference on Information Literacy (ECIL)*, p. 102. Retrieved from https://helda.helsinki.fi//bitstream/handle/10138/300381/ecil2018bookofab-stracts.pdf?sequence=1#page=132, accessed 7 Oct. 2019.

Chapter 15: Money Matters

Cancer Research UK [no date]. Tobacco control local policy statement. Retrieved from https://www.cancerresearchuk.org/sites/default/files/tobacco_control_local_policy_statement.pdf, accessed 7 Oct. 2019.

European Centre for Monitoring Alcohol Marketing, 24 Mar. 2014. New research: End-of-aisle displays associated with increased alcohol sales. Retrieved from http://eucam.info/2014/03/24/new-research-end-of-aisle-displays-associated-with-increased-alcohol-sales-2/, accessed 7 Oct. 2019.

George, M., 31 May 2019. Exclusive: Data reveals poor pupils' Xmas jumper shame. *TES*. Retrieved from https://www.tes.com/news/exclusive-data-reveals-poor-pupils-xmas-jumper-shame, accessed 7 Oct. 2019.

McNeill, A., Gravely, S., Hitchman, S. C., Bauld, L., Hammond, D. and Hartmann-Boyce, J., 2017. Tobacco packaging design for reducing tobacco use. *Cochrane Database of Systematic Reviews*, (4). doi:10.1002/14651858. cd011244.pub2.

NHS, 31 Dec. 2017. Help for problem gambling. Retrieved from https://www.nhs.uk/live-well/healthy-body/gambling-addiction/, accessed 7 Oct. 2019.

Chapter 16: Better Problem-Solving

National Offender Management Service, Sep. 2015. Working with offenders with personality disorder: A practitioners [sic] guide. Retrieved from https:/ /www.england.nhs.uk/commissioning/wp-content/uploads/sites/12/2015/10/ work-offndrs-persnlty-disorder-oct15.pdf, accessed 7 Oct. 2019.

Chapter 17: How Therapy Can Help

British Psychological Society, Oct. 2017. Memorandum of understanding on conversion therapy in the UK. Retrieved from https://www.bps.org.uk/sites/ bps.org.uk/files/Policy/Policy%20-%20Files/BPS%20Memorandum%20 of%20Understanding%20on%20Conversion%20Therapy%20in%20 the%20UK%202.PDF, accessed 7 Oct. 2019.

Royal College of Psychiatrists, Mar. 2018. Racism and mental health. Retrieved from https://www.rcpsych.ac.uk/pdf/PS01_18a.pdf, accessed 7 Oct. 2019.

Sankar, A., Melin, A., Lorenzetti, V., Horton, P., Costafreda, S. G. and Fu, C. H., 2018. A systematic review and meta-analysis of the neural correlates of psychological therapies in major depression. *Psychiatry Research: Neuroimaging, 279*, pp.31–9. doi:10.1016/j.pscychresns.2018.07.002.

Chapter 18: Making Change Stick

Jędrzejczyk, J. and Zajenkowski, M., 2018. Who believes in nonlimited will-power? In search of correlates of implicit theories of self-control. *Psychological Reports*, p.0033294118809936. doi:10.1177/0033294118809936.

The limits of lifestyle
The Health Foundation, Mar. 2018. What makes us healthy? An introduction to the social determinants of health. Retrieved from https://www. health.org.uk/sites/default/files/What-makes-us-healthy-quick-guide.pdf, accessed 7 Oct. 2019.

World Health Organization [no date]. Social determinants of health. Retrieved from https://www.who.int/social_determinants/sdh_definition/en/, accessed 7 Oct. 2019.

Final Word: Are You a Policymaker?

Gesch, C. B., Hammond, S. M., Hampson, S. E., Eves, A., & Crowder, M. J., 2002. Influence of supplementary vitamins, minerals and essential fatty acids on the antisocial behaviour of young adult prisoners. *British Journal of Psychiatry*, 181(01), 22–28. doi:10.1192/bjp.181.1.22

Acknowledgements

To my clients past and present, thank you for entrusting me with the privilege of helping you. Your courage and commitment is inspiring. I learn from you every day.

To Francesca Zampi and Harry Grenville, my managers, and the whole family at FOUND for being, frankly, outrageously good at your jobs. Honestly, look at what you've created! This agency has helped me to push towards the boundaries of my potential and there is still more to come! Shona Vertue – I owe you a drink or two.

To the dream team at Yellow Kite. To Nicky Ross, Rebecca Mundy, Emma Knight, Caitriona Horne and Holly Whitaker, for seeing the potential in the book, recognising the urgency of the message and supporting me as a first-time author. Your genuine enthusiasm for the book and your incredible work in shaping and building the project helped to erase any lingering doubts I might have had about whether I really had anything interesting to say.

To the researchers whose tireless and sometimes thankless work is the foundation of my own thinking, clinical practice and this book. Thank you for all that you do to improve the lives and health outcomes of millions. I hope I have done your efforts justice.

To the wonderful people who read my posts on Instagram, participate in the Thinking Space Book Club, listen to the Stronger Minds podcast and come to events. Thank you for your time and energy. You are all quite wonderful.

A big thank you to The Glitch Mob, John Legend, Mariah Carey, Drake, Sounds of Blackness, Labi Siffre and the late Amy Winehouse, whose music either powered me through a writing session or emboldened my spirit when I began to feel overwhelmed by the task and responsibility of writing a book like this.

Index

everyday emotion management 200–2
limbic system and 32
logic and 39
relationships and 206
stress inoculation 208
tough love and emotional resilience 288
understanding 31, 32–3, 173–203
emulsifiers 126–7, 315
endocannabinoids 38, 148
endorphins 38, 148, 226
endowment effect 260
envy 188–90
essential fatty acids 97–8, 103
European Food Safety Authority 125
evidence-based medicine (EBM) 18–23, 24
exercise 65, 143–61, 208, 212, 223, 225

Facebook 16, 239–40, 241–2, 307
failure: dealing with 219–22
    mistaken belief that mental illness is sign
        of 279
faith, drawing on 210–11
fake news 248–52, 253–4
fasting 133–42
fats, saturated vs unsaturated 97
fibre 108, 110, 111, 121, 132
fight or flight response 36, 38, 186
Finnish Geriatric Intervention Study to
    Prevent Cognitive Impairment and
    Disability (FINGER) 300–1
fish, oily 97–9, 117, 118, 121, 131, 132
FODMAPS 152–3
foetal alcohol syndrome 122–3
folate 101
food: fasting 133–42
    food frequency questionnaire 91–4, 97
    foods to limit 122–8
    improving brain health through 90–132
FOXO3 137
Frankl, Viktor 214
Freud, Sigmund 191
friendships 206–7, 222
fructose 124
fruit 131
funding, mental health research 11
future discounting 294–5, 301
Future Self, saying hello to 302–3

gambling 260–2, 263
Gambling Commission 260
gamma-aminobutyric acid (GABA) 38
generalised anxiety disorder (GAD) 33–4
ghrelin 136
Gibson, Belle 16, 248
glia 28, 39
global disease burden, mental illness and 7–13
glucose 123–4, 130, 132, 133, 136
glutamate 38
gluten 128–9
glycogen 136
glymphatic system 71, 227
go-betweens, children as 289
goals 215, 301
Graham, Paul 251
greens, leafy 101–3
grief 220
guilt 193–5
the gut: emulsifiers and 126
    gut barrier junction 111
    gut-brain axis 112
    gut microbiome 108–13
    immune system and 131
    polyphenols and 114
    sweeteners and 125

habits 231–2, 304
Haidt, Jonathan 207–8
Hamilton Depression Rating Scale 17
    (HDRS17) 164
handwriting notes 246–7, 253
healthy eating index 94–5
heat 224–9, 237
heat shock proteins (HSPs) 227, 228
herbs 105–7, 132
hippocampus 33
    Alzheimer's disease and 35
    BDNF and 146
    depression and 34
    GAD and 34
    meditation and 230
    neurogenesis 50, 98, 136
    physical activity and 146, 147
    power of mantras on 167
    smells and 167, 168
    stress and 59, 60
histamine 43

About the Author

Kimberley Wilson is a nutrition trained Chartered Psychologist. Her clinical work looks at the role nutrition and lifestyle play in mental health, including disordered eating, functional disorders of the gut-brain axis and our emotional relationships with food. Her private London clinic, Monumental Health, provides a comprehensive approach to mental health treatment, combining psychological therapy with nutrition and lifestyle support.

books to help you live a good life

Join the conversation and tell
us how you live a #goodlife

🐦 @yellowkitebooks
📘 YellowKiteBooks
📌 Yellow Kite Books
📷 YellowKiteBooks

ROGERSTONE

20.3.20